W9-AVS-701

THE NEW
BODY TYPE
GUIDE

GET HEALTHY, LOSE WEIGHT & FEEL GREAT

THE NEW BODY TYPE GUIDE

GET HEALTHY,
LOSE WEIGHT
& FEEL GREAT

FORMERLY
**THE 7 PRINCIPLES
OF FAT BURNING**

Eric Berg, DC

KB PUBLISHING | ALEXANDRIA, VA

Limit of Liability/Disclaimer of Warranty

KB Publishing Inc.
P.O. Box 11716
Alexandria, VA 22312

For more health information from Dr. Berg, visit www.DrBerg.com.

To my beautiful wife, Karen, and my
fantastic children, Jordan, Allison and Ian,
for putting up with my being so often in the
"cave" office, behind the computer screen.

Contents

1. Missing Link—the Educational Step 1

2. The 7 Principles of Fat Burning 5

The Purpose of Food 5

Principle #1

There Are Four Different Body Shapes,
Each Influenced by Hormones 8

Principle #2

Calories Are Insignificant Compared
to Fat-Burning Hormones 10

Principle #3

You Have to Be Healthy Before You Can Lose Weight 12

"My Hormone Blood Tests Are Normal" 13

What Is Fat? 14

Principle #4

Environmental Hormones and Chemicals
Mimic Your Hormones 16

Principle #5

You Have to Heal Your Glands and Hormones
to KEEP the Weight Off 17

How Do You Know It's Working? 19

Principle #6
*Fat-Burning and Fat-Storing Hormones
Have Their Own Triggers* 19

Principle #7
Incorrect Exercise Prevents Fat Burning 20

The Exercise-Longer-to-Lose-Weight Myth 21

Sticking to a Diet 21

3. Hormones and Your Body Shape 23

What Is a Hormone? 24

Gland-Hormone Connection 25

What Causes Gland and Liver Problems? 26

GMO 30

Anti-fat-making-hormone Foods 31

Coffee 32

Fat-Burning and Fat-Storing Hormones 33

Fat-Burning Hormones 33

Growth Hormone (GH) 33

Insulin-like Growth Factor (IGF) 33

Glucagon 34

Adrenaline 34

Thyroid Hormones (T3 and T4) 34

Testosterone 34

Fat-Storing Hormones 35

Insulin 35

Estrogen 35

Cortisol 35

4. Finding Your Body Type 37

Take the Quiz to Find Out Which Body Type You Are! 37

The Body Type Quiz 37

Why Am I a Mixed Type? 41

5. The Adrenal Type 43

The Adrenal Glands 43

The Adrenal Type 45

Adrenal Deficiency 52

Causes of the Adrenal Body Type 65

Adrenal Type Symptoms 66

6. The Ovary Type 69

The Ovaries 69

The Ovary Type 70

Causes of the Ovary Body Type 72

The Menopause Backup Organ 73

Ovary Type Symptoms 75

7. The Thyroid Type 77

The Thyroid Gland 77

The Thyroid Type 78

The Sluggish Thyroid 79

High Cholesterol
   Are You Sure It's Really Genetics or Eating Fatty Foods? 82

The Thyroid Problem Is Usually Secondary 86

Causes of the Thyroid Body Type 88

Estrogen 89

Cruciferous Vegetables and Iodine 91

If You Are Missing Your Gallbladder 91

Thyroid Type Symptoms 92

8. The Liver Type 93

The Liver 93

The Liver Type 95

Causes of the Liver Body Type 103

Testing for Liver Damage 105

Creating a Healthy Liver 106

Cholesterol and Eggs 107

Atherosclerosis 108

Liver Spots 108

Growth Hormone 109

Key Indicators 111

Liver Type Symptoms 113

9. The 10 Fat-Burning Triggers and Blockers **115**

Trigger #1: The Absence of Sugar 116

Trigger #2: Vegetables 121

Examples of Shakes I Consume 124

Cruciferous Vegetables 125

Trigger #3: Protein 126

Trigger #4: Fats 129

Satisfying Effect 131

Two Types of Fuel 131

Hungry Cells That Can't Eat 133

Essential Fats 133

Trans Fats 134

Saturated Fats 135

Trigger #5: Skipping Meals and Intermittent Fasting 136

Trigger #6: Gland Destroyers 138

Alcohol (beer, wine or mixed drinks) 138

Caffeinated Products (coffee, soda, tea and chocolate) 139

Drugs 140

Detoxification 140

Growth Hormones 141

Endocrine Disruptors 141

Food and Cosmetic Chemicals 142

Consuming Food without Enzymes 142

Trigger #7: Water Retainers 143

Trigger #8: Exercise 145

Trigger #9: Stress 146

Trigger #10: Sleep 147

   Eating before Bed 148

   Nutritional Supplementation and Sleep 148

10. Fat-Burning Strategies **149**

What Is Insulin? 150

Intermittent Fasting 152

Insulin Index 154

   Insulin Resistance 155

Polycystic Ovarian Syndrome 157

High Blood Pressure 157

   What Spikes Insulin 157

Corrective Actions 158

   Keep Your Sugar at Zero 158

   Add More Fat 158

   No Snacking 158

Additional Tips 159

   Apple Cider Vinegar 159

   Exercise 159

   Potassium 160

   Vitamin B₁ 162

   Sleep 162

   Stress 162

   Medications 163

11. Step ONE: Basic Eating Plan **165**

Overall Summary 166

Strengthening Your Digestive Weaknesses 167

   Bloating 167

   Indigestion 168

   Acid Reflux, Heartburn (or GERD) 168

Constipation 168
　Special Note on Your Gallbladder 169
Irritable Bowel Syndrome (IBS) 170
General Overview 171
Rules 171
　Other Examples of Hidden Sugars 172
Breakfast 172
Lunch 173
Dinner 174
Food Intake 174
Unlimited Vegetables 174
Dairy 176
Don't Eat Starches 176
Don't Eat Grains 177
Allergies and Food Sensitivities 177
Salad Dressings 177
Fruits 177
Animal Proteins 179
Fish (wild-caught) and Seafood 180
Grass-Fed, Organic Meats 180
Eggs 181
Vegetarian Proteins 181
Fats 181
Raw Nuts and Seeds 182
　Pecans 183
Beans/Lentils/Legumes 186
Supplement Intake 186
Apple Cider Vinegar & Lemon Drink 187
Symptoms of pH Imbalance 188
A Few Guidelines 188
Three-Day Sample of What to Eat 189
Quick Healthy Small Meals 190
Salad Ideas 191

Concentrated Nutrition 191

What to Expect 192

What's the Next Step after Two Weeks? 193

12. Tailor-Making Your Eating to Your Body Type **195**

Adrenal 196

Dietary Proteins 196

Dietary Fats 196

Nutrients 196

pH and Your Adrenals 197

Stress-Reducing Techniques 197

Exercise 198

Liver 198

Dietary Proteins 198

Dietary Fats 198

Carbohydrates 199

Nutrients 199

Liver Technique 199

Ovary 200

Dietary Proteins 200

Dietary Fats 201

Nutrients 201

Thyroid 202

Dietary Proteins 203

Dietary Fats 203

Nutrients 203

Thyroid Technique 204

How to Know If Things Are Working 204

Insulin Resistance Improvement 204

Hypoglycemia (low blood sugars) and Dietary Protein 204

Basic Rules of Eating for Hormone Health 205

Avoid sugar, fruits, grains and starches 205

Consume lots of nutrient-dense vegetables 206

Hunger between meals 206
Consume the right amount of protein for your body type 207
Consume the right amount of fat for your body type 207
Avoid gland blockers 207
Avoid fluid retainers 207
Get your sleep 208

13. Additional Eating Information **209**

So-Called Natural Foods 209

Sugar and Hidden Sugars 210

Gland Blockers 212

Water Retainers 213

Beverages 213

Mercury in Fish 215

Clarification on Protein 215

Eggs—the Perfect Food 216
Omelet Ideas 218

14. Sticking to It—GUARANTEED! **219**

Temptation 219

Stress Eating 219

Discouraged by No Results 220

Craving Sweets 221

Eating out of Boredom 221

Eat Everything on Your Plate? 222

Rewarding Yourself with Food 222

Social Situations or Eating Out 222

More Tired on the Plan 223

Constipated on the Plan 224

Vivid Dreams 224

15. Body Issues That Interfere with Losing Weight 225

   Fatigue 226

      Injury Technique 226

   Sleep Problems 227

   Poor Cognitive Function (Memory) 227

   Low Stress Tolerance 228

   Cravings for Carbs or Sweets 228

   Inflammation 229

   Menstrual 230

   Hot Flashes 230

16. Ridding Your Body of Stress 231

   Massage Tool 232

      Rules for Use 232

   Quick Overview 233

   The 7 Stress Points 234

      #1 Upper-Neck Points 234

         How Does It Work? 235

      #2 Occipital Points 235

      #3 Mid-Neck Points 237

      #4 Lower-Neck Points 238

         How Does It Work? 239

      #5 Mid-Back Points (Static and Dynamic) 239

         How Does It Work? 241

      #6 Collarbone Points 241

      #7 Adrenal Points 243

17. Exercising for Your Body Type 245

   Exercising but Still Can't Lose? 245

   Exercise Doesn't Burn Fat: It Triggers Fat-Burning
Hormones to Burn Fat 246

Basic Principles of Exercise and Hormones 247

    Calories and Muscle Mass 248

    Calories Are Insignificant Compared to Hormones 249

    Eating Before, During or After 249

    Rest between Exercises 249

    Sleep Quality and Amount 249

    Stress Level 250

The Difference between the Body's
Two Main Energy Systems 250

The Aerobic Energy System
Low Intensity—Longer Duration 250

The Anaerobic Energy System
Higher Intensity—Shorter Duration 252

Liver/Thyroid Body Type Exercise Plan 253

    Use Anaerobic Only 253

    The Benefits of Anaerobic Exercise 254

    Caution about Anaerobic Exercise 254

The Hormone Connection to Exercise 255

    Intensity and Difficulty 255

    Frequency 256

    Duration 256

    Types of Exercise 256

    Rest and Recovery 257

    Plateau 257

Hormones Triggered by Anaerobic Exercise 258

    Anaerobic Exercise Routine 259

Adrenal Body Type Exercise Plan 263

    Use Aerobic 263

    The Benefits of Aerobic Exercise 263

    Working Harder Will Initially Slow Your Progress 263

    Aerobic Exercise Routine 264

    Don't Stop Before You Start Burning Fat 266

    History of Long-Term Sugar Consumption 266

Ovary Body Type Exercise Plan 267
    Use Aerobic and Anaerobic 267
Summary 267

18. Enjoy Good Food! **269**
Some of Dr. Berg's Favorite Recipes 269
Healthy Pleasure Foods 283
Milkshake Alternative 304
Soda Alternatives 305
Alcohol, Wine and Beer Alternative
    Kombucha Tea 306
Acceptable Alternative Flours 306
Chocolate Alternatives 307
Acceptable Sweeteners 307

19. Questions and Answers **309**

Acknowledgments 325

Glossary 327

References 343

Bibliography 347

Resources 351

Index 357

Conscious Eating Cards (cut-out) 379

1

Missing Link—the Educational Step

Have you ever felt that it shouldn't be so hard or take so much effort to lose even a little bit of weight? Well, the last thing you need is another diet! If you are simply told what to eat and it doesn't work for you, you'll chalk up a loss and go on to the next diet, creating further losses, and then think there is a problem with you, that you have poor willpower (an inability to stick with something).

Working with thousands of individuals has led me to believe that people really do *not* have a problem with willpower—they simply have never been taught the right way to lose weight. No one is going to stick with a program that's not working. But if you do the correct thing and *you know how to do it*, it *will* work and you will stick with it.

In my clinic, I have found that the missing link is an educational step. Once a person has the background and understanding of HOW fat is burned and HOW health is created, they succeed. But if you simply tell them what to do, you've done nothing for them of any lasting value.

There are so many weight-loss books out there that say, "Scientific studies have shown . . ." or "Everyone knows . . ." or "Experts say . . ." That type of approach is very far from conveying understanding.

This book is different.

I want to help you solve a big problem—stubborn weight. To do that, we must first make sure we have identified the *correct* problem. Many people are attempting to fix the wrong problem: their weight (which is actually the symptom). You also need to know what controls metabolism—hormones—because you are going to use these hormones to work for you instead of against you. Hormones are chemical messages produced by glands. You have six fat-burning and three fat-making hormones, and each is triggered by different things. Might it not be a good idea to know *what* these are and *how* to trigger them?

The New Body Type Guide is not necessarily for people who can lose weight easily; it is for those who have a very stubborn metabolism. *The New Body Type Guide* gives you the most effective leverage over weight loss because it addresses the very things that control weight loss—fat-burning hormones. To my knowledge, no other book in existence gives you an easy-to-understand summary of how to use food and activities to trigger all of your fat-burning hormones. Most people don't even know these exist, let alone how to get them to work.

Fat is not a cushion or insulation, as many people think, but is a store of reserve energy, and I'm about to show you how to get your body to tap into and run on this energy. Most people are running their bodies on sugar fuel and rarely use fat fuel, yet right now you already have within your own body everything you need in order to tap into your fat reserves.

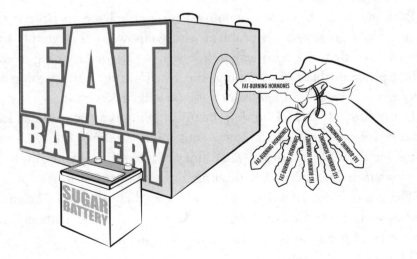

You are going to be triggering not just one hormone but *all* six key hormones to create maximum fat-burning effects. As a result, you not only WILL lose major weight but will get extremely healthy at the same time. The nice thing is that some of these hormones are anti-aging as well.

Different bodies need different solutions. I have found that most people fall into four different types and need different variations of food (especially protein) and exercise. In chapter 4, you'll be taking a quiz to find out which body type you have. Once you start the eating plan, you'll soon find out what your body responds to best in order to lose the most weight possible in the shortest period of time with the least effort.

What you might not have realized is that your own hormones have been working against you, making you fat and distorting your body's shape. Instead of giving you the same old same old, I'm going to help you find out which hormone or gland is responsible for your body type and guide you to the best program to fix the problem.

You will be eating nutrient-dense foods, which will knock out cravings for sweets, breads, salty snacks and chocolate and keep you satisfied.

Everyone will start with the Basic Eating Plan given in chapter 11. Based on your results, you will then tweak things to fit your primary body type; however, I recommend giving yourself two weeks on the basic plan before tweaking anything.

If you are consistently losing weight and the results are good, you will stay on the basic eating plan but enhance your progress with some minor changes based on your body type. The secret is to align your actions with your body type until the results are consistent. If we know what gland in your body is not operating at 100 percent, then we can enhance it and enhance your weight loss too. In the previous edition, you were directed to start with the Liver Enhancement, then move to your body-type eating plan. When I realized that the idea of a mixed body type created confusion for some people, I changed our approach to make it simpler: we start with a more basic plan, then add more complex solutions if needed.

This is a lifestyle change, not just a diet you do to lose weight and then go back to junk foods. It has been our experience that as people increase their health, their bodies no longer desire refined sweet foods but crave nutrient-dense whole foods.

Anyone can lose weight on just about any diet. The most unique and exciting thing about this program is that you will be able to keep the weight off because you are correcting the cause. With this program, you will be stabilizing the glands and hormones that have been responsible for making you fat in the first place. If you simply do what everyone else is doing—losing the weight without fixing the cause of the problem—the weight will just come right back. Your primary goal needs to be getting your weakest gland healthy so that you can stay permanently at your ideal weight.

The absolute maximum fat a person can burn per week is two pounds. However, water weight can come off at two to five pounds per day in some cases. In one extreme case, I had a patient eliminate a full bladder of fluid 12 times within a 24-hour period. So, how much water weight or fat weight you have will determine how quickly you will lose the weight. But the problem you've been running into is that your own hormone system has been blocked, preventing your body from burning fat and from losing water weight. Our goal is to fix this problem and keep you in fat-burning mode throughout this entire process.

Your energy will be significantly increased and your sleep will become much sounder and deeper; your digestion will improve and your nails, skin and hair will also be in better condition, because hormones control these body activities and characteristics. Many of my patients have lowered cholesterol and blood pressure on this program as well.

Through a study of this book you will identify your own body type and learn some fascinating things about how your body works and how it stops working, especially in regard to fat burning. The idea is to teach you how to look beyond diets and exercise and instead use hormone triggers from foods and exercise. This way you will never have to depend on a program but will be in full control of your own weight and health. Nobody will have to tell you what to eat at a social gathering or a restaurant because you yourself will be able to tell the difference between what causes fat and what burns fat.

We are talking about the thing that you live in—your body—and since you do live inside it, it might be of benefit to understand the owner's manual.

2

The 7 Principles
of Fat Burning

Many people have been trying to lose weight with various diet and exercise programs. Everywhere you look you see another diet popping up—cabbage soup, cookie, peanut butter, grapefruit, high-protein, etc. I want you to take another route. I want you to understand what's behind a stubborn and resistant metabolism before you jump into the solution.

You're about to benefit from my 29 years of working with tens of thousands of people.

The clinic at my Northern Virginia Health & Wellness Center has been an excellent testing ground where we have helped thousands of different types of patients, using diet, exercise and nutrition. My current focus, in order to expand my ability to help a larger group of people, is on educational YouTube videos, online membership sites, and remote health coaching. My online Exclusive Membership site provides a variety of health solutions that range from nutrition and healthy eating to my acupressure techniques for body types.*

My approach has consistently been a teaching one, and I always like to start with the fundamentals of good health. Which brings us to the next topic: the purpose of food.

The Purpose of Food

A main confusion many people have is with the very definition of *food* and its purpose. They think of it as "something you eat to get pleasure, to reward

---

* For information on the Exclusive Membership site, see Resources section.

and treat yourself with." But in no dictionary could I find this definition. Check out the following definition from the *Macmillan Dictionary*:

Food *n*. that which is eaten to sustain life, provide energy, and promote the growth and repair of tissues; nourishment [Old English *fōda*, "nourishment"]

According to this definition, a lot of people are living on something other than food. Let me tell you what I do when I am shopping at the grocery store or eating at a restaurant. I ask myself several questions: Is this an imitation of food or a man-made food-like substance? Will this substance ADD more life, more health, and will it nourish and repair my tissues, or will it reduce my health?

The question now becomes, how do we classify or know which foods are really foods and which are non-foods? What substances are essential to life? What substances can we not live without? What is the body made out of, which if missing will create illness?

The vital substances necessary to the body are referred to as "essential"—as in *essential amino acids* and *essential fatty acids*. *Essential* means "cannot be made by the body and MUST come from the diet." Amino acids, for example, are the building blocks that make our hair, nails, eyes, muscles, joints, etc. Fatty acids make up the outer and inner structures of our cells, not to mention our brains, nerves and hormones.

There are many nutrients that if missing from the body will cause disease. These essential raw materials must also include vitamins and minerals. And enzymes must be added to this list because consuming foods that are void of enzymes can create degenerative diseases. Enzymes are the things that do the work of the body, similar to assembly workers in a factory.

Foodstuffs that contain all of these nutrients are more *food* than those that leave out these factors or contain them but in a destroyed or altered form, as happens when food is cooked, pasteurized, processed or roasted. Simply stated, foods containing all these factors—amino acids, fatty acids, vitamins, minerals and enzymes—and in an optimum balance would create the most health. This is why isolated food factors such as those in protein shakes (isolated soy protein), synthetic vitamins (petroleum derivatives), refined sugars and carbohydrates (which have to be enriched with synthetic vitamins because they are depleted) are more *non-foods* than anything else. So, we have a scale from healing foods to illness-creating non-foods. This book is about consuming foods that naturally contain all five building blocks. I have also created more than 2,000 YouTube videos (over 78 million views) teaching how the body works, with tips you can implement to make your own body super healthy. I have organized these videos on my blog at DrBerg.com.*

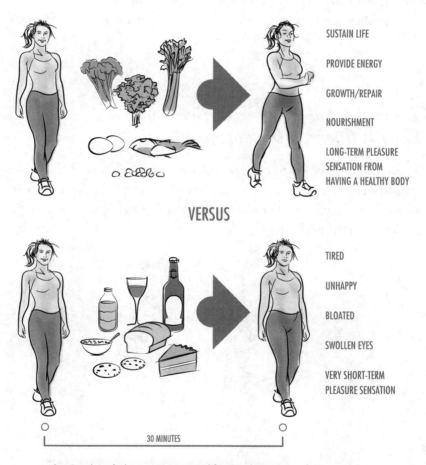

food *n.* that which is eaten to sustain life, provide energy, and promote the growth and repair of tissues [Old English fōda, "nourishment"]

The word *diet* also has an interesting derivation.

Diet *n.* a regulated course of food and drink to promote health or for weight control—*v.i.* to eat according to prescribed rules [Old French *diète*, from Latin *diaeta*, "**way of living**"]

---

* Dr. Berg's blog: https://www.drberg.com/blog.

Diet stems from the word meaning "a way of living"—which is an interesting new viewpoint compared to the older idea of "something people do to deprive and starve themselves."

By understanding and then applying this broader concept of eating and living to create health as you go through this program, you WILL end up with the byproduct of a slim, healthy body.

The following are the seven key principles on which our program is based.

Principle #1

There Are Four Different Body Shapes, Each Influenced by Hormones

You might have heard of pear and apple shapes but probably not what's behind these distortions. Certain hormones have the purpose of directing where fat is placed on the body, and it is a distortion of this function that causes different body shapes.

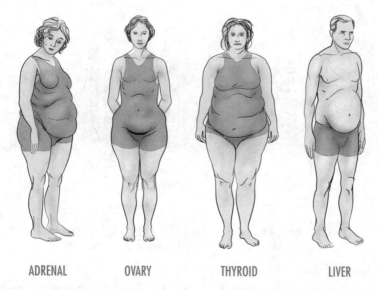

| ADRENAL | OVARY | THYROID | LIVER |

As mentioned earlier, the primary purpose of fat is not to be a cushion or insulation. Its primary purpose is to provide an alternative fuel source when we run out of sugar fuel. In other words, fat is the alternate fuel used when there is no more sugar available.

In truth, our original fuel source in the olden days was fat. Our bodies did very well on fat fuel, and we have the cellular machinery for this as well. Fat is a cleaner, more efficient and more stable fuel, enabling you to avoid the highs and lows of blood sugar fluctuations. Running your body on fat instead of sugar could be compared to running your car on electricity versus diesel fuel.

But your body will ALWAYS use sugar first as a priority. Only when the body is depleted of dietary sugar will it switch back to fat fuel—the key words being *depletion of sugar*. Even tiny amounts of sugar can block fat burning. This is why you must keep sugars at zero. Zero. Sorry. But don't worry; there's some good news coming—you WILL be able to consume sweet desserts, just not desserts made from actual sugar.

The other trigger that will prevent fat burning is stress. Stress activates hormones to keep you in sugar-burning mode; and even if there is no sugar in the diet, the body can turn its own proteins (muscles) into sugar. More on this later.

I've been on a mission for many years to find the real underlying causes of health problems and stubborn weight, and I think you are going to like what I have found.

The distinctive quality of this program is the discovery that different body shapes are the result of specific correlating glandular problems (adrenals, ovaries, thyroid and liver). This program targets ALL of these problems, allowing for maximum weight loss. One can't just put everybody on the same foods and expect to be successful. Each person needs to eat and exercise for his or her specific gland weakness.

I have identified *four* different and distinctive types of weight problems.

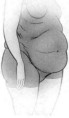 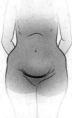 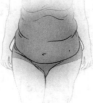 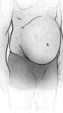

| ADRENAL | OVARY | THYROID | LIVER |
| SAGGING/HANGING | SADDLEBAGS | WEIGHT ALL OVER | PROTRUDING POTBELLY |

The outside of the body gives clues as to what's going on inside. In the case of the adrenal glands, the body when under stress will store energy (as fat) around the vital organs—in the abdomen. If there is an ovary problem, you'll see excess fat accumulate around the hips and thighs with a lower-stomach bulge just under the bellybutton. When there is a weakness in the thyroid gland, because thyroid hormones are directed into all cells of the body, an overall appearance of weight gain will occur rather than in just one location. And when the liver is weak, fluid can leak into the sac around the abdomen, giving a "potbelly" appearance.

The Adrenal body shape is adipose tissue surrounding the organs in the abdomen (intra-abdominal fat) and is called a pendulous abdomen. The Latin derivation of *pendulous*, the verb *pendere*, means "to hang or sag." The Ovary body shape is more of an estrogen cellulite-type fat, which is superficial (just under the skin) and mostly below the bellybutton. People call this "saddlebags" with a lower-stomach bulge. The Thyroid body shape is yet a different type of fat altogether. The weight is deposited all over the person's body and is not really fat but more of a waste-like substance that accumulates between the cells. This condition is known as myxedema, and it can be likened to a sponge that holds in liquid and will not release it. *Myx-* comes from the Greek word *myxa*, meaning "mucus" or "slime," and *edema* comes from the Greek *oidēma*, which means "swelling." Then there is the Liver body shape. This is not always a fat situation; it can be a fluid problem, where an accumulation of fluid is leaking into the abdomen.

You'll learn about these body types in detail in chapters 5 through 8.

Principle #2

Calories Are Insignificant Compared to Fat-Burning Hormones

You have probably been told that weight gain or obesity is caused by "consuming more calories than are burned" and the way to lose weight is to eat fewer calories. That is what I once believed too. But how do we explain the skinny guy who eats like a horse yet doesn't gain an ounce? And what about the overweight person who looks at food across the table and gains five pounds?

The real problem lies more in metabolism and the hormones that control it. When you cut calories, you can initially lose weight. But then it rebounds and you will gain back more later, especially in the stomach area, because "low calories" or "hunger" is the trigger for the fat-storing stress hormone. We'll get into that later.

Calories are units of energy in various foods.

Hormones look at food calories differently. Without having a good understanding of hormones, it might appear that *all* calories are the same and if you eat less you will of course weigh less. People who tell you this have not grasped the basic physiology of hormone interaction resulting from foods. And the obvious proof of this is that you probably have been cutting calories with minimal or no effect. A theory is only as true as it works.

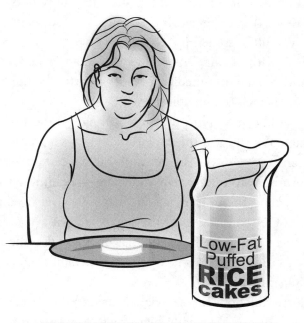

FAT-MAKING HORMONES LOOK AT CALORIES DIFFERENTLY

Even though fats have the densest calories, they are neutral when it comes to making fat. Sugar and refined carbohydrates, on the other hand, are huge triggers to fat-making hormones despite having fewer calories than fats. And although protein has calories, consuming the right amount of protein will trigger fat-burning hormones. The "right amount" is based on your body type, which I'll explain later in this book.

Principle #3

You Have to Be Healthy Before You Can Lose Weight

You have no doubt heard that you should lose weight so you can be healthier, because obesity is a health risk causing heart disease, diabetes, arthritis and stroke. Right? People have been pushing the idea that *fat* directly causes these other problems.

This is not true!

I found it is just the opposite. You need to be healthy first before you can actually lose weight. You are fat because some area of your body is unhealthy. In other words, heart disease, diabetes, arthritis, stroke AND obesity are all the result (symptoms) of the same thing—an unhealthy body. Somehow, someone has assigned *obesity* as a primary cause or a disease, when in reality it is an effect or result of something else.

The problem with making it a disease is now it gets treated with medication, and if some non-medical practitioner treats it, he or she could be practicing medicine without a license.

If you have stubborn weight problems, you have unhealthy hormones. You can't be fat and healthy at the same time.

The body can't and won't release fat until it is at a certain level of health. It shouldn't surprise you to learn *why* your body is holding on so dearly to fat if you understand the purpose of fat. It is a survival mechanism, and the body will not let go of fat until the sugars are not available anymore. Interestingly, sugar can come from the diet or it could come from stress. Stress triggers a hormone, cortisol, which has the ability to convert body proteins into sugar fuel.

You could force your body to lose weight by taking an appetite suppressant, drinking canned diet shakes with high-fructose corn syrup or starving yourself; but this would not be the optimum solution, as it would give you a bigger problem down the road. Jumping in and fixing your weight problem with dieting (cutting calories) and typical exercise, without first finding out *what* problem you have, would not be the best approach either. Losing weight would be a lot more difficult because you'd be focusing on the wrong goal—weight loss. The correct goal is to create healthier glands and hormones. The weight loss will then occur as a benefit of having a healthier body.

So here is what I want you to change, right now. From now on, NO LONGER TREAT SYMPTOMS!

Your weight is a symptom, not the cause. Shift all your energy and attention to fixing the cause by creating a healthy body and the symptom of weight *will no longer be a problem*. Can you imagine an auto mechanic spending his entire time trying to cover up the clanking sound in the engine of your car? We've applied this principle to thousands of people and it works every single time.

This brings up the next question: Which foods have the capacity to create the greatest health for your body?

Let's first take the reverse of that: What condition is the most unhealthy? The answer, of course, is cancer. And are there foods that could potentially inhibit or reverse cancer? Yes sir! Anti-cancer foods would be the healthiest foods you could possibly eat to create health and burn fat. These would be cruciferous vegetables, including kale, broccoli, Brussels sprouts, cabbage, radish and others.

I think the entire concept of an unhealthy gland or hormone causing a distorted body has been given little attention for this one reason: Many doctors base their entire diagnosis on blood tests. These are fine for diagnosing major disease states but not for detecting subclinical gland and hormone imbalances. You have to have major liver damage before positive findings show up on blood tests. The same is true of the adrenal glands.[1] Your body tends to keep the blood chemistry constant no matter what.

"My Hormone Blood Tests Are Normal"

I can't tell you how many times I've heard, "My hormone blood tests came out normal but I have all the symptoms and I'm still fat." Let me explain something. Rarely are the relationships between the hormones looked at. For instance, if the adrenals overproduce their stress hormones, the important fat-burning hormone—growth hormone—can be suppressed. If your ovary has a cyst on it, excessive estrogen can be produced, which can block the thyroid and create thyroid symptoms (hair loss, overweight, brittle nails, etc.).

---

1. This and other numbered references throughout the chapters can be viewed in the References section, beginning on page 343.

Eighty percent of thyroid hormone activation occurs through the liver, so a person with thyroid symptoms could have normal thyroid hormones but have liver damage; and failing to look deeper at the relationship between these two organs, the person's focus could be on the wrong problem and they could end up trying to resolve a secondary situation for years with no success.

So, if you have problems yet tests keep coming out normal, ask your doctor to evaluate more broadly. If you only check the thyroid hormones, you can miss the adrenal, ovary or even the pituitary hormones. Without really evaluating the hugely significant importance of hormone interactions, a person is stuck "treating the symptoms."

But please realize I am not an endocrinologist, and this book is not about diagnosing or treating any medical disease or condition. It is more an education to inform you how your body works, with emphasis on the fat-burning effects of hormones through food and exercise. I believe it is important to inform people how their own bodies work, since the word *doctor* means "teacher."

Excess fat is a symptom, simply the tip of the iceberg, not the actual cause. You could say the most important discovery has been that the majority of people are attempting to solve the wrong problem. Have you ever tried to solve the wrong thing? This leads to wasted time and energy with no results!

Let's take a look at the real problem—the failure of your fat cells to release energy. To solve this problem, you need to first know what a fat cell is and its purpose.

What Is Fat?

Though not commonly realized, fat is the largest endocrine gland in the body. Being an important part of body composition, adipose tissue (fat) accepts a lot of hormonal signals and is able, as well, to produce and secrete hormones and hormone-like substances.

Fat contains potential energy. *Potential* means "capable of being or becoming; possible but not actual." Fat is potential energy because it is fuel that has not yet become energy. It is stored energy or reserve energy.

The truth is you're not really *fat*; you just have too much potential energy. Sounds better, doesn't it? You should get a T-shirt that says, "I'm not FAT. I have lots of POTENTIAL ENERGY"!

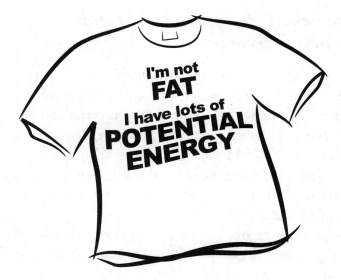

Fat is similar to money in the bank. You go to work every day and produce something for your paycheck. You then pay your bills; anything extra goes into your bank account. Hopefully you don't spend everything you make and you have some extra reserves in the bank. You have access to this money through an ATM card, credit card or your bank account number and proper identification. Fat is equivalent to the body's reserve bank account. I know what you are saying right now: "I must be a billionaire!"

But how could you have all this extra potential energy and at the same time be even the slightest bit tired? You might even crave energy—in the form of breads, pasta, cereals, chips or chocolate. It's a weird situation—having tons of stored potential energy, yet you can't release it. That is because this stored energy is *unavailable* to you. You need a specific key to release the fat and turn it into energy. Well, guess what? You already have the keys; they are your own hormones. To do this, though, you have to understand these keys and use the right ones. You have roughly 600 hormone keys. Of this number, six are fat-burning and three are fat-storing. If any of the three fat-storing hormones are active, they will nullify ALL six fat-burning hormones. The secret is to activate the six and keep the three inactive.

Principle #4

Environmental Hormones and Chemicals Mimic Your Hormones

If you want to know why your weight problem is becoming worse, you don't have to look far. You are presently being exposed to synthetic environmental hormones on a daily basis. The meats and meat products we eat come from animals that have been given hormones—chickens, turkeys, cattle and fish. Certain groups will tell you there is no proof that these man-made hormones administered to animals have any effect on our bodies. Yet if you go overseas to countries that don't use these hormones, people are thinner—Europeans especially.

Another interesting observation is that chemicals such as pesticides and insecticides have the ability to act like hormones in our bodies. Your food is heavily sprayed with these toxic chemicals.

The Environmental Protection Agency has a name for these chemicals; collectively they're called *endocrine disruptors*, meaning any chemicals that mimic, block or otherwise disrupt the normal function of hormones.

I talked to a Russian cab driver recently while being taken to the airport. I asked him, "Are people in Russia fat compared to Americans?" He said, "No, I've never seen so many fat people in my life since moving to America. In Russia, you only see someone fat with some sort of sickness." In Russia, he used to be a driver for a chicken factory, so I asked him if they use growth hormones to grow chickens as they do in America. He said no and replied that they just keep the lights on and provide lots of food for the chickens and they keep eating 24/7. He said, "You Americans have restaurants and food places open when you should be sleeping—and Americans are like those chickens that can't stop eating." I then asked him about drinking vodka, because I was curious about damage to the liver. I wanted to know if Russian people have protruding bellies, and, sure enough, he said they do. The Liver body shape shows up as a potbelly.

Principle #5

You Have to Heal Your Glands and Hormones to KEEP the Weight Off

The aim of this book is to change your viewpoint of the primary goal from losing weight to complete healing of your weak gland—achieving stable weight loss. Let's focus on the real problem!

The key to keeping the weight off is achieving full rejuvenation of your glands and hormones—in other words, doing the program long enough for your body to fully heal. Not completely fixing the true problem (unstable glands) causes the problem to come right back.

When certain glands get sick, the hormones they produce can physically dissolve the muscles in your legs, buttocks and arms, leaving you with shrunken, weak and flaccid muscles. These destructive hormones literally eat up muscle proteins, turning them into fat around your midsection. So, instead of using fat reserves for fuel, your body uses muscle proteins, which are turned into sugar as fuel, leaving you fat, flabby, stressed and weak.

As a person starts the program and these glands heal, the muscles need to be rebuilt. These muscles are a bit heavier than fat; therefore, the person's weight might not initially change, even though their clothes feel looser. Before the body will burn fat, it has to build back this lost muscle tissue.

> I had a female patient who was over 350 pounds. In the first month she didn't lose any weight at all, yet her energy, sleeping, digestion and muscle strength were greatly improved. Most people would be discouraged by this, since they'd be looking at the weight indicator only. In my mind she was right on track, because the second month she lost 23 pounds, and by the third month she had lost a total of 61 pounds. Her body had to grow protein in her leg muscles before burning fat, and protein weighs more than fat.

I have found that fat will come off in direct relation to the health of your hormones. Because fat, to the body, is survival (reserve energy), the body will not release this energy until it is sure it's in safe mode. As can be seen in the following diagram, while healing is occurring it might take some time before your body is healthy enough to burn fat and lose weight. It could take about a month before the weight starts to come off. However, your energy will be up, you'll feel stronger, have fewer cravings, and your overall mood will improve.

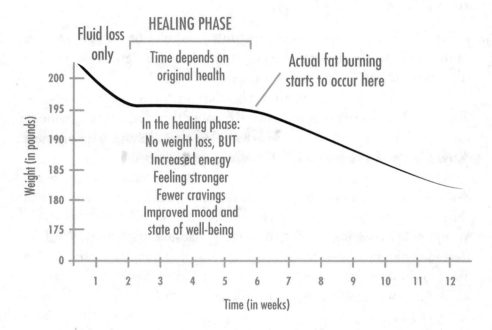

Adipose tissue is *only* used when absolutely necessary—after the sugar fuel has been exhausted. The body *always* uses stored sugar or dietary sugar as a priority before tapping into fat fuel. This is the principal reason why people are not losing weight. Most of them are running their bodies on sugar fuel. You must deplete your sugar reserves BEFORE you can tap into your fat reserves.

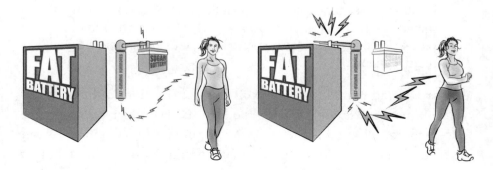

How Do You Know It's Working?

The best way to know if your organs and glands are healing and the program is working is not just by weight loss but by other positive health indicators—improved energy, better quality of sleep, better digestion, clothes fitting more loosely, more muscle strength, better nail and hair quality, decreased cravings, and overall feelings of well-being. These indicators give you the valuable feedback that your body is healing.

In other words, you need to shift your goal from "losing weight" to "attaining health," since only through this can you fully reach your ideal weight, as overweight is a symptom of an unhealthy body.

It's amazing what obese people are fed in certain obesity clinics— powdered sweet chocolate mixtures with very low calories, diet pills, appetite suppressants and B$_{12}$ shots. They will experience a very temporary weight reduction, but these treatments will bring a person's health downward in the long run.

> A woman came to my clinic with constant burping after consuming one of these powdered mixtures. Burping means gallbladder and liver problems. It's one thing to not have a successful weight-loss program, but it's another thing to worsen the entire situation.

Principle #6

Fat-Burning and Fat-Storing Hormones Have Their Own Triggers

Hormones control metabolism and each one associated with fat burning and fat storing has its own triggers. Hormones are triggered or blocked by foods, exercise and other activities.

There are two things that can happen with these triggers. You can eat and exercise to stimulate fat burning or you can eat and exercise for fat storing. The huge hidden problem I discovered was that most people are nullifying the fat-burning hormones by using the wrong triggers. For instance, correct exercise might work if you can get seven hours of quality sleep per night, whereas poor or inadequate sleep will prevent fat burning.

And just a little bit of sweet carbohydrate can set your fat burning back for a day. This is why "everything in moderation" doesn't work with fat burning. Another example is drinking wine at night, as alcohol is a gland (liver) destroyer and can set back fat burning for hours or days.

The more of these hormone triggers you implement correctly, the faster and easier weight loss will be. Therefore, instead of wasting time counting calories, use the hormone triggers.

You will learn all of these important triggers in detail in chapter 9.

Principle #7

Incorrect Exercise Prevents Fat Burning

Another key discovery has been that different body types need different kinds of exercise.

I'm sure you have heard the theory "You're fat because you just don't exercise enough." Well, if you have an Adrenal body type and you do hard-core exercise, you not only will prevent fat burning, your body might even get bigger. I see these people at the gym with their personal trainers working to lose weight for years with very little change. Exercise only works if your body has good adrenals. If you have an Adrenal body type, adding more exercise to an already stressed-out body is self-defeating. Adrenal types need very light, slow exercise.

On the other hand, if you have a Liver body type, the fat-burning hormones need to be stimulated intensely for weight loss to occur. If the exercise is too light or too slow, you get no effects. Exercising for your specific body type can be a big advantage in maximizing weight loss.

Many people have the idea that their fat is excess calories and all they need to do is burn these off through exercising. However, it's not the calories burned during exercise that are significant. It's the delayed fat-burning peaks that occur between 14 and 48 hours later[2]—but only if specific conditions are correct in regard to sleep and stress levels.

The Exercise-Longer-to-Lose-Weight Myth

This philosophy is currently being pushed heavily in gyms. I have had quite a few patients come to my office who were exercise enthusiasts. One woman not only was exercising two hours per day seven days per week but she also ran a 26-mile marathon—with *zero* weight loss. Talk about depressing!

Since the adrenals are the stress glands, if you have an Adrenal body shape, then the longer and harder you exercise, the less you will lose because you are triggering those darn stress hormones again—causing more belly fat.

So, there is a specific way you should be exercising to trigger fat burning, depending on your specific gland weakness. In chapter 17 you will learn exactly how to exercise for your body type.

Sticking to a Diet

This entire book could be summarized as teaching you how to get into and stay in healthy fat burning.

One of the greatest challenges for most individuals is sticking to a diet program once started. There is a very important reason for this. If you were to lose only two pounds a week from a diet, you might become discouraged and discontinue, especially if your friend down the street lost eight pounds per week. Fat loss unfortunately does not occur as quickly as fluid loss. But, on a positive note, many people have lots of water weight to lose, and losing that alone can hugely change the way someone looks. It might even be possible to lose six pounds of water weight per week for several weeks; but as soon as your water weight becomes normal, the weight loss for a person with a healthy metabolism is one to two pounds per week. If you don't know this, you can easily give up.

3

Hormones and
Your Body Shape

The hormonal system as a whole is called the endocrine system. If you look up the word *endocrine*, you will find it comes from *endo-*, a combining form that means "within" or "inner," and the Greek word *krinein*, which means "to separate." *Webster's New World Dictionary* then says, "see CRISIS." When you go to the word *crisis*, you find it comes from the same derivation, "to separate, discern." This is interesting because the endocrine system IS the system that discerns or determines threats to normal survival, keeping the body out of crisis via hormones.

If its survival is threatened in any way, the body will start to hold energy—which is the accumulation of fat. This is the body's attempt to keep you alive and surviving; and as long as the threat to survival remains, fat will be held on to tightly and will overdevelop to compensate for the lack of survival.

Many people think that the shape of a body is purely genetic and there is nothing that can be done about it. It is true that there are genetic tendencies. It is also true that hormonal imbalances will cause excessive distortions of accumulated fat in different locations around the body. An imbalance on the inside can show up on the outside.

Hormones do diminish as you age, but that is not the sole reason for your weight problem. Take a look around—younger people are getting fat too. Some of the fat-burning hormones are also the anti-aging hormones. So the goal of this program is twofold: to help you lose weight and to make you younger.

The hormone system is very sensitive to environmental chemicals, especially growth hormones in the foods we eat. Our foods are injected with hormones; they are also sprayed with pesticides, which have the ability to mimic hormones. You have been swimming in a sea of toxic chemicals. Welcome to planet Earth!

When these chemicals enter the body, they plug up or interfere with hormone receptors. Glands make and send hormones. Cells then receive these in a similar way to a catcher in a baseball game. If you are born with 20,000 hormone receptors per cell and are constantly exposed to environmental growth-hormone mimickers—chemicals such as pesticides and insecticides—eventually these block the receptors, leaving very few for hormone reception. It's like driving into New York City and trying to find a parking place. As you age, the chemical exposure accumulates until your system gets overwhelmed and can't burn fat anymore. But it's not just older people; young people get fat too due to this environmental toxicity factor.

What Is a Hormone?

A hormone can be defined simply as a chemical message produced by a gland in the body and sent through the bloodstream to another area where it causes some effect. For example, exercising can create fat-burning effects that last for 48 hours after the workout. There are over 600 different hormones in the body, each with a unique function. Fat burning, fat storing, appetite, sleep, hair and fingernail growth, fluid levels and joint repair are just a few examples of direct effects that hormones have on the body.

Hormones are the language of the body. Instead of words, hormones tell the body what to do, causing millions of effects each day. Glands create these messages; they both send and receive communications. Daily functions of the body are controlled mainly by hormones; for instance, they tell the heart how fast to pump and the bones how quickly to grow. If hormones become dysfunctional, a person could have osteoporosis (thinning of the bones) despite the amount of calcium consumed.

Each gland has its own purpose in regulating certain areas of the body. The adrenals, for instance, help the body to handle stress in all its different aspects. Imagine for a moment a person starting to slip on some water while stepping down a flight of stairs. The adrenal glands would send off adrenaline (stress-response hormone), which would put the body in high gear and prepare it for intense stressful action. Or imagine if you accidentally stepped on a large rattlesnake in your backyard. Your adrenal hormone adrenaline would spike, increasing the heart rate, creating sensations of fear, and pumping out instant energy to ready the body to hightail it out of there!

Gland-Hormone Connection

There is always a two-way connection back and forth within a properly working hormonal system. Not only do the glands talk but the cells of the body's tissues need to be listening as well. Once a message is sent and received, the cells are supposed to send a message back to let the gland know that the request has been received and complied with.

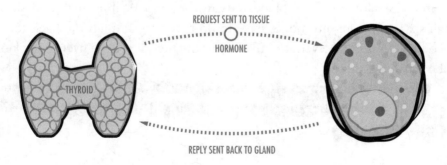

REQUEST SENT TO TISSUE

HORMONE

THYROID

REPLY SENT BACK TO GLAND

The word *communication* is derived from *common*, which means "shared equally." In order to have good communication you need an equal balance (50-50) of talking and listening. Hormone messages need to be received before they can work. If the receptors (mini-ears) within the body are blocked, there is no connection—similar to attempting to communicate to someone with earplugs.

The gland is giving the command or order "BURN FAT," and the fat cells are saying, "I'm sorry, did you say something?" And if the fat cells are not listening or are not receiving messages from the gland, no fat burning occurs.

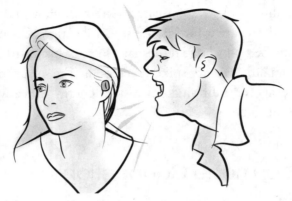

Or what about the person who talks so much that you tune them out? If because of a lack of response the gland starts "talking" too much, the fat cells eventually begin ignoring the fat-burning hormone messages.

Each gland, when in trouble, will create very specific bodily symptoms—the most noticeable one being a reshaping of the body. It takes years in some cases for hormone blood tests to show up as abnormal; and since all six fat-burning hormones have to do their job through the liver, there could be a normal level of hormones in the blood, yet the liver might not be activating them.

No matter how much you starve yourself, no matter how hard you exercise, if the fat-burning hormones are not being triggered, there will be no weight loss.

What Causes Gland and Liver Problems?

I've made some interesting observations with regard to why Americans are overweight. In Northern Virginia where I practice, I have a melting pot of patients from all over the world. Upon surveying people from other countries, I have almost always found that they started becoming overweight when they moved to America. Some have told me that they lost weight when they went back home despite calorie intake or fat in their diets. This led me to evaluate the differences and similarities between America and other countries. Yes, people in other countries consume fewer fast foods and eat more fresh and natural foods, but they don't seem to be eating fewer fatty foods or lower-calorie foods. They might also be getting more exercise; but then again, despite getting plenty of exercise, many Americans are not able to lose weight. So we can't just blame it all on "You're eating too much," or "You're not exercising," or "You're getting old."

What is the big difference or the real common denominator?

There is one significant factor I'd like to discuss. In America we fatten cattle, chickens and other animals via hormones. We give them estrogen and growth hormone to make them fatter. Even farm-raised fish are fed hormones. Well, if you consume turkey meat from turkeys that have been given hormones from birth, is it possible that some of the residue from the hormones could leach out in your body? If hormones can cause turkeys to look butterball size, is it possible that your body could also become butterball size?

Due to the presence of hormones in our food supply, we are seeing girls develop larger breasts and start their menstrual cycles at an increasingly younger age. Young boys are even developing extra breast tissue. This alone tells us that estrogen levels must be higher. Young girls with excessive sex drives may also have been exposed to estrogens in their diets.[1] Growth hormone, used in animal foods such as commercial milk, seems to be having an effect on our children as well—bigger feet especially. And I have observed women gaining weight when they go on the birth-control pill or on hormone replacement therapy—again more estrogen.

Estrogen makes the fat layer around a female body. Fat cells also produce estrogen. Estrogen can inhibit thyroid and liver function.

Don't worry—it gets worse!

The Environmental Protection Agency (EPA) is doing major research on the effects of toxins called *endocrine disruptors* in both humans and wildlife.[2]

An endocrine disruptor is an environmental poison that mimics, blocks or otherwise disrupts the normal function of hormones.

Examples of endocrine disruptors are

- pesticides: pest killers

- insecticides: insect killers

- herbicides: weed killers

- fungicides: fungus killers
- plastics
- solvents
- heavy metals

(The suffix *-cide* comes from the Latin word *caedere*, which means "to kill.")

The EPA has found that 90–95 percent of all pesticide residues are found in meat and dairy products.[3]

These chemicals act as if they were hormones. They have the ability to interfere with the binding of hormones. If hormones are keys and cell receptors the keyholes, endocrine disruptors can fit into these holes

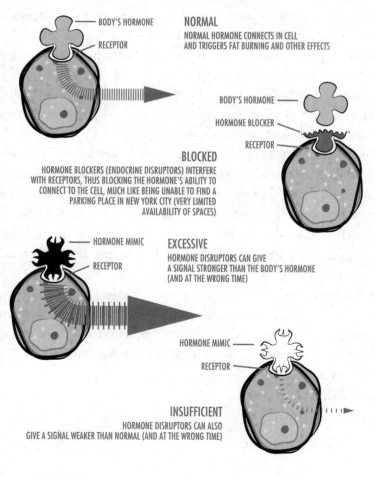

METHODS OF HORMONE MISCOMMUNICATION

BODY'S HORMONE
RECEPTOR

NORMAL
NORMAL HORMONE CONNECTS IN CELL
AND TRIGGERS FAT BURNING AND OTHER EFFECTS

BODY'S HORMONE
HORMONE BLOCKER
RECEPTOR

BLOCKED
HORMONE BLOCKERS (ENDOCRINE DISRUPTORS) INTERFERE
WITH RECEPTORS, THUS BLOCKING THE HORMONE'S ABILITY TO
CONNECT TO THE CELL, MUCH LIKE BEING UNABLE TO FIND A
PARKING PLACE IN NEW YORK CITY (VERY LIMITED
AVAILABILITY OF SPACES)

HORMONE MIMIC
RECEPTOR

EXCESSIVE
HORMONE DISRUPTORS CAN GIVE
A SIGNAL STRONGER THAN THE BODY'S HORMONE
(AND AT THE WRONG TIME)

HORMONE MIMIC
RECEPTOR

INSUFFICIENT
HORMONE DISRUPTORS CAN ALSO
GIVE A SIGNAL WEAKER THAN NORMAL (AND AT THE WRONG TIME)

and block our hormones from functioning. Over time as a person ages and accumulates exposure to these chemicals, the receptors that are supposed to receive hormones get plugged, reducing hormone communication. This explains why hormones can lose their effectiveness and become resistant or stubborn. In other words, the key (hormone) can't fit into the keyhole (receptor) anymore.

Another point regarding endocrine disruptors is that even tiny amounts can create hormone damage. It doesn't take much.

Schools, restaurants, golf courses, yards, foods, etc., are sprayed with chemicals that mimic estrogen. These toxins usually accumulate in only one or two organs.[4]

"Really?"

Yes...

des PLEX®

to prevent ABORTION, MISCARRIAGE and PREMATURE LABOR

recommended for routine prophylaxis in ALL pregnancies . .

96 per cent live delivery with desPLEX in one series of 1200 patients*— — bigger and stronger babies, too.*

No gastric or other side effects with desPLEX — in either high or low dosage***

* * * * TIMES ■ SATURDAY, MAY 22, 2004   **13A**

Pesticides persist in Americans' bodies

ATLANTA — A comprehensive survey of more than 1,300 Americans has found traces of weed and bug killers in the bodies of everyone tested, leading environmentalists to call for far tighter controls on pesticides.

The survey, conducted by the U.S. Centers for Disease Control and Prevention, found that the body of the average American contained 13 of these chemicals.

A surprising finding was that 99 percent of Americans, including virtually all children born in recent years, had DDT residues. The use of the insecticide has been subject to controls and outright bans since the late 1960s, and its presence indicates how persistent it is in the general environment.

Between 1938 and 1970, doctors prescribed an artificial estrogen named diethylstilbestrol, or DES, to prevent miscarriages in millions of pregnant women. It was not until 30 years later that doctors discovered that DES had caused miscarriages, a rare form of cervical cancer, and many other health-related problems. One round of DES was equivalent to over 5,000 birth-control pills. This was also the main growth hormone being given to animals during the same time.

DDT, another chemical that mimics hormones, was found to be stored in the fat tissues of over 99 percent of children (May 22, 2004) despite being banned in 1969. Where is this coming from? We are allowed to sell it to third-world countries such as Mexico and Chile. Take a wild guess where we purchase our fruits and vegetables in the winter months.

These endocrine disruptors are also carcinogens. If you read any textbook on toxicology (study of poisons), you'll find these terms are synonymous. Carcinogens are those substances capable of causing cancer.

The word *cancer* has an interesting history. The cancer first found by the Greek physician Hippocrates was breast cancer, and the blood vessels that spread around the breast looked like crab legs; hence the Greek derivation *karkinos*, meaning "crab."

The reason you probably haven't heard much of this information broadly promoted is because it's difficult to prove. Carcinogens usually have a latency period of 30 or more years after initial exposure before tumors or cancer is observed. This is why it took 30 years to show up in daughters of mothers who took DES. These chemicals accumulate insidiously in certain tissues over the years, and since they compete with your hormones, the hormonal effects become less and less and the hormones can't quite connect to do their function.

GMO

GMO means "genetically modified organism." A genetically modified organism is a plant or animal whose DNA (cell blueprint) has been modified without using natural methods of reproduction. Individual genes are transferred from one organism into another organism. This produces crops that carry certain traits such as resistance to insect damage and herbicides (chemical weed killers).

As an example, in the case of genetically modified corn, genes from a bacterium that carries a trait making it resistant to herbicides are inserted into the plant. As a result, the corn crop can withstand herbicides.

Monsanto, the main company that produces GMO seeds, also sells Roundup, Monsanto's brand-name herbicide containing a chemical called glyphosate. Many GMOs, such as soy, corn, beet sugar, canola and alfalfa, are designed to be resistant to the effects of Roundup. These patented breeds of plants are known as Roundup Ready because they make it possible for farmers to get away with spraying the herbicide on their crops in order to kill weeds without killing the crops.

Monsanto states that "trillions of GMO meals" have been consumed in the United States without any adverse effects. However, there are no human studies and only a few very short-term (three months) animal studies, and the great majority of these were done by Monsanto itself.

A longer-term independent animal study (performed by a French scientist named Gilles-Éric Séralini) on GM food did show some serious negative effects, such as triggering tumors, organ failure, gastric lesions, liver damage, kidney damage, allergic reactions and more. Unfortunately, this study was retracted from publication, something which almost never happens. This tells you how powerful Monsanto is politically.

The Séralini team reported that 50 percent of male rats and 70 percent of female rats died prematurely, compared with only 30 percent and 20 percent in the control group.

Monsanto has major political power, which has influenced labeling laws—laws that now prevent us from knowing if GM ingredients are present in our foods. The only way you can control this is to make sure you consume organic foods or eat foods that say "Non-GMO." But you can be pretty confident that most of the soy and corn is genetically modified.

Avoid GMOs if at all possible, because presently we are all going through a human experiment, and unfortunately the true damages will not show up until years after these companies have made their billions.

Anti-fat-making-hormone Foods

The food plan I will be explaining later in the book has as one of its goals reducing in your food supply chemicals that mimic estrogen (fat-making hormone). Certain foods increase estrogen and others decrease it. There's one group of foods that is anti-estrogen and anti-toxin, called cruciferous (cabbage, broccoli, cauliflower, radish, kale, Brussels sprouts, etc.). *Cruciferous* comes from the Latin word *crux*, meaning "cross," since the flowers of these vegetables are shaped like a cross. If we're dealing with chemicals in the body, it makes sense to consume as many of these vegetables as possible or take them in whole-food supplement form.

To make a natural cleaning fluid for washing vegetables, mix one-third of a cup of apple cider vinegar in a gallon of water. This will remove some superficial chemicals, although nothing can remove the internal chemicals. Also, break off and discard the outer leaves of leafy vegetables.

Trim the fat from meat and the skin from poultry and fish if they are commercial. Also, if given a choice between commercial fish and commercial meat, go for the fish. It takes 60 pounds of pesticide-sprayed feed and hay to produce 1 pound of edible beef, not to mention growth hormones given throughout the lifetime of the cattle. It takes only 1 pound of feed to produce 1 pound of edible fish—hence fewer hormone-disrupting chemicals.

Coffee

Drinking two cups of coffee each day means buying some 18 pounds of beans each year—the total annual yield of 12 coffee trees. To keep those trees productive, coffee farmers apply 12 pounds of fertilizers and pesticides every year. Even though this program is going to recommend not drinking coffee, during the transition period I recommend consuming organic coffee. Coffee also contains caffeine and is damaging to your adrenal glands, a factor that can keep you from burning fat.

Organic means without the use of chemical fertilizers, pesticides, fungicides, herbicides and insecticides. When you read labels, you want to make sure they say "Organic," not "Natural." These are not the same.

Natural, in legal terminology, only means that those foods are not treated with chemicals during processing. *Natural* can mean many different things but it doesn't mean without pesticides or insecticides. I'm not saying you have to start eating 100 percent organic foods tomorrow. However, I would recommend eating at least 50 percent organic foods.

Now, you are not going to go to your friend's house for dinner and say, "You know, um . . . I recently read Dr. Berg's book, and um . . . I noticed that that meal you're about to serve me is filled with pesticides, insecticides, herbicides, heavy metals, antibiotics and growth hormones. . . . And that tuna has mercury in it. . . . I hope you don't mind—I brought my own food in this bag here." You wouldn't do that; it's not socially accepted—you'd never be invited over again. Maybe that's why no one invites me to dinner anymore.

Fat-Burning and Fat-Storing Hormones

In order to understand the fat-burning hormones that trigger weight loss, you might want to know what these are. The following list gives not only the fat-burning hormones but also the fat-storing hormones, which you want to avoid triggering.

Fat-Burning Hormones

Growth Hormone (GH)

Growth hormone is made by a gland in your brain called the pituitary. Once made, it travels down to and works through the liver. This is a fat-burning, lean-muscle-building hormone. One of its key functions is building up cartilage and collagen. Without growth hormone, your joints and muscles fall apart and you age more quickly, as it's also an anti-aging hormone. GH regulates fuel between meals and is active as well during the night while you sleep. Poor liver function affects GH function. It is stimulated by protein and intense exercise. Interestingly, it is *not* triggered by light exercise.

Insulin-like Growth Factor (IGF)

IGF is made by the liver and is triggered by growth hormone. Its basic function is giving the body fuel between meals, and it does this through releasing stored sugar and fat; thus it is a fat-burning hormone. Insulin is the opposing hormone to control body fuel while you are eating, whereas IGF is stimulated when the stomach is empty. When the liver is damaged, this hormone decreases, putting added stress on the pancreas to supply fuel through raised insulin.

Glucagon

Glucagon raises blood sugar by tapping into the fat reserves and is therefore called a fat-burning hormone. It has an opposing action to insulin. It helps control blood sugar between meals and is stimulated by dietary protein and intense exercise. However, if excess protein is eaten, insulin will be elevated and will blunt this hormone.

Adrenaline

Adrenaline is the main hormone that releases fat from the fat cells. It has many additional functions to prepare the body for stressful situations: mental alertness, increased heart rate, metabolic rate, blood pressure, etc. It is triggered by exercise.

Thyroid Hormones (T3 and T4)

These hormones control the speed of your metabolism. They trigger metabolism by increasing the size and number of the cellular energy factories, called mitochondria. The faster the metabolism, the thinner the person is. People with insufficient thyroid hormone secretion are overweight. One way to inhibit these hormones is to cut calories and deprive your body of nutrients.

Testosterone

Testosterone is made by the adrenal glands, the testicles, and even the ovaries. This fat-burning hormone assists in giving you lean muscles and is involved in sex drive and male characteristics. If a female has high testosterone, she gets facial hair, a deeper voice and male-pattern baldness. It is stimulated by exercise and countered by estrogen.

Fat-Storing Hormones

Insulin

Insulin is made by the pancreas; its function is to lower blood sugar after meals. It will cause the cells to absorb sugar as fuel and will convert the rest to fat and cholesterol. Insulin works with IGF and glucagon to keep fuel constant in the blood; so when IGF and glucagon go down, insulin must go up and vice versa. In the presence of insulin, you will not be able to burn fat. Sugar triggers insulin. Large amounts of protein can trigger insulin. The more lean or low-fat a protein is, the more insulin is released. And lastly, eating triggers insulin. This is why "two to three meals without snacking" is very good advice if you want to not only lose weight but also improve diabetes.

Estrogen

(From the Greek word *oistros*, meaning "mad desire," + *genēs*, " born")

Estrogen is responsible for the female characteristics, menstrual cycle and changes of the uterus and breasts. It provides the fat layer around a female body, especially around the outer thighs. The reason women tend to have more fat than men lies in the fact that women have over a thousand times the concentration of estrogen receptors that men have.

Cortisol

This is an important hormone produced by the adrenal glands, which is activated by stress of all kinds. It is anti-inflammatory and releases sugar from the liver and muscles into the blood as an instant fuel source for stressful events. Cortisol is classified as a fat burner; however, it also has an indirect fat-storing effect when it turns body-muscle proteins into sugar fuel, since this forces insulin to deal with the excess sugar in the bloodstream, producing weight gain in the midsection.

4

Finding Your Body Type

Take the Quiz to Find Out Which Body Type You Are!

Each body type has its own characteristics. Taking this quiz helps to zero in on your specific type. You might find, as you do the quiz, that you answer yes to questions in more than one body type and so think, "I'm mixed between a few types." This could be true, but there is always a primary; most people have a primary type that is causing secondary symptoms. One type can create problems for another type, as you will learn in the last section of this chapter. When one hormone increases, others can decrease. The purpose of this quiz is not to diagnose you. The purpose is to inform you about your body and help to find possible areas of weakness based on how glands behave when they are stressed.

The Body Type Quiz

Before you do the complete quiz, there are several questions upfront that will quickly find out if the liver and gallbladder are involved. If the answers to these questions are yes, then your body type is most likely a primary Liver type.

If you answer YES to ANY of the seven points below, you do not need to go through the quiz—you already have your answer.

	YES	NO
1. Have had your gallbladder removed	❏	❏
2. History of gallstones	❏	❏
3. Can't lose weight on high-protein diets (e.g., Atkins)	❏	❏
4. Dislike consuming lots of heavy protein-type foods	❏	❏
5. Inability to digest fatty or greasy foods, especially at night	❏	❏
6. History of liver problems	❏	❏
7. Protruding, distended belly—potbelly	❏	❏

DIRECTIONS: Circle one letter (A, B, C or D) in each question below. If there is more than one symptom that you are experiencing within a question, circle the one that is most prominent.

For women who are menopausal or post-menopausal, the Ovary (D) questions should be answered from the viewpoint of having had, or not had, previous problems with or a history of the condition mentioned.

1. Do you . . .	A. crave sweets, breads and pasta?	a. Thyroid
	B. crave salt (pretzels, cheese puffs or salty peanuts) or chocolate?	b. Adrenal
	C. crave deep-fried foods or potato chips?	c. Liver
	D. crave ice cream, cream cheese, sour cream or milk?	d. Ovary

2. Are you . . .	A. often depressed or feeling hopeless?	a. Thyroid
	B. a worrier or often anxious and nervous?	b. Adrenal
	C. irritable, moody, grouchy, in the morning?	c. Liver
	D. moody/irritable at certain times of the month?	d. Ovary

3. Do you . . .	A. feel better on fruits and berries?	a. Thyroid
	B. need coffee or stimulants to wake up?	b. Adrenal
	C. experience a tight feeling over your right lower-stomach area or rib cage?	c. Liver
	D. experience constipation during menstruation?	d. Ovary

4. Do you have . . .	A. brittle nails with vertical ridges?	a. Thyroid
	B. facial hair as a female?	b. Adrenal
	C. pain/tightness in right-shoulder area?	c. Liver
	D. pain in right or left lower-back/hip area?	d. Ovary

5. Do you have . . .	A. a weight problem more evenly distributed?	a. Thyroid
	B. a pendulous abdomen, meaning hanging, sagging and loose?	b. Adrenal
	C. a protruding abdomen (potbelly)?	c. Liver
	D. excess fat on thighs and hips (saddlebags) and a lower-stomach bulge?	d. Ovary
6. Do you have . . .	A. dry skin, especially hands and around elbows?	a. Thyroid
	B. swollen ankles—socks leave creases on ankles?	b. Adrenal
	C. flaky skin or dandruff in eyebrows and scalp?	c. Liver
	D. menstrual cyclic hair loss?	d. Ovary
7. Do you have . . .	A. indentations on both sides of your tongue where the tongue meets the teeth?	a. Thyroid
	B. atrophy (shrinkage) of the thigh muscles with difficulty getting up from a seated position?	b. Adrenal
	C. dark yellow urine?	c. Liver
	D. hot flashes?	d. Ovary
8. Do you have . . .	A. a loss of hair on the outer third of the eyebrows?	a. Thyroid
	B. dizziness when getting up too quickly?	b. Adrenal
	C. hot or swollen feet?	c. Liver
	D. menstrual cyclic brain fog?	d. Ovary
9. Do you have . . .	A. to sleep with socks on at night because of feeling cold?	a. Thyroid
	B. chronic inflammation in body?	b. Adrenal
	C. headaches or head feels heavy in morning?	c. Liver
	D. excessive menstrual bleeding?	d. Ovary
10. Do you have . . .	A. puffiness around eyes?	a. Thyroid
	B. an unusual feeling of being "out of breath" while climbing stairs?	b. Adrenal
	C. skin problems (psoriasis, eczema, brown spots)?	c. Liver
	D. low sex drive?	d. Ovary

11. Do you have . . .	A. excessive skin sagging under arms?	a. Thyroid
	B. twitching under or on top of left eyelid?	b. Adrenal
Are you . . .	C. not a morning person, yet feel more awake at night?	c. Liver
Do you have . . .	D. weight gain one week before menstrual period?	d. Ovary
12. Do you . . .	A. have dry hair and hair loss?	a. Thyroid
	B. wake up in the middle of the night (2:00–3:00 a.m.)?	b. Adrenal
	C. have a deep crevice (deep crease appearance) down center of tongue and/or a white film on tongue?	c. Liver
	D. have an upper body which is thinner than your lower body?	d. Ovary
13. Do you experience . . .	A. not being able to maintain curls in your hair after using a curling iron?	a. Thyroid
	B. cramps in the calves at night?	b. Adrenal
	C. more itching at night?	c. Liver
	D. water retention at certain times of the month?	d. Ovary
14. Do you . . .	A. become excessively tired in the early evening (7:30–8:00 p.m.) and more awake in the early morning?	a. Thyroid
	B. have a more active bladder at night than during the day?	b. Adrenal
	C. have a yellow tint in the whites of your eyes?	c. Liver
	D. have a history of ovarian or breast cysts?	d. Ovary
15. Do you have . . .	A. a lack of get-up-and-go (vitality)?	a. Thyroid
	B. calcium issues or deposits—bursitis, tendonitis, kidney stones, heel spurs, early cataracts?	b. Adrenal
	C. major moodiness if you skip a meal?	c. Liver
	D. difficulty losing weight after pregnancy?	d. Ovary

16. Do you have . . .	A. a history of being on low-calorie diets?	a. Thyroid
	B. low tolerance for stressful situations, get easily irritable and on edge?	b. Adrenal
	C. stiffness and pain more in the right shoulder and right side of neck?	c. Liver
	D. pain and tightness in one knee, worse during menstrual cycle?	d. Ovary

Count up the total of each:

Total A. Thyroid ___8___   Total B. Adrenal ___12___

Total C. Liver ___122___   Total D. Ovary ___2___

The letter with the highest total indicates your primary body type. Knowing this, you will be able to both enhance your eating plan in chapter 12 and follow the correct exercise plan in chapter 17.

If you were not able to clearly determine your body type from this quiz, look through the symptoms listed for each body type at the end of chapters 5, 6, 7 and 8 to see which symptoms you have the most of—Adrenal, Ovary, Thyroid or Liver.

Why Am I a Mixed Type?

As mentioned earlier in the chapter, most people have a primary problem and many secondary issues. For instance, an overactive ovary can inhibit the thyroid, creating weakness and symptoms in the thyroid, yet the real problem is in the ovary. If the liver is blocked, the thyroid is automatically inhibited because 80 percent of thyroid function occurs through the liver. If the adrenal glands are overworking and producing excess hormones, growth hormone from the liver will be inhibited, which will force the pancreas to produce more insulin, causing increased fat in the abdomen. So you can see the complexity of these relationships and the importance of finding the root cause.

5

The Adrenal Type

The Adrenal Glands

You have two adrenal glands, one located on top of each kidney.

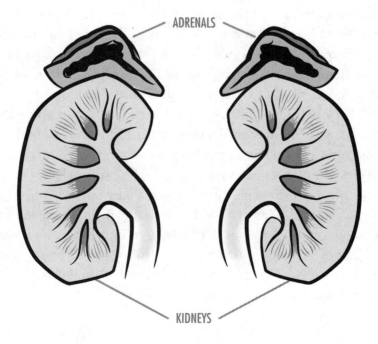

THE ADRENAL GLANDS

One of the main functions of these glands is countering stress by the production of several hormones. The adrenals don't know the difference between physical and mental stress; they treat both with the same stress hormones. Every type of stress influences these glands[1]—injury, infection, divorce, financial stress, job-related stress, irritable people, drugs and medication, surgery, pain, illness, poison ivy, extreme cold or heat, giving birth, menstrual cycle, staring into computer monitors, eating junk foods, starvation diets, and babysitting 15 small children under the age of five for over 13 hours.

The adrenals have many other functions, from anti-inflammatory actions (ridding the body of pain and swelling) and immune system protection to balancing fluid and salt levels, and controlling minerals (such as potassium), rapid heart rate and sleep and awake cycles. They even act as backup organs for the ovaries during menopause.

The following is a description of what happens when the adrenal glands do not function properly.

The Adrenal type I am about to describe is the result of excessive adrenal hormone production. I will cover adrenal hormone deficiency as well.

Excess fat in both the midsection (buffalo-like torso) and the face can occur from overreaction of this gland. In the midsection, the fat forms primarily in and around the abdominal organs and sags downward over the belly. Another term for this stomach is *pendulous*, meaning "hanging loosely," "sagging." This is different from the Liver body shape, which is a potbelly or a protruding stomach like a water balloon, while in the Ovary body shape the person has a small bulge below the bellybutton.

The majority of Americans hold weight in the stomach area more than any other place (which could come from the adrenals or the liver). There are different degrees of adrenal problems, but many of them do not show up on blood tests until they are well advanced into dangerous stages. The adrenal glands are set on a timing mechanism in the brain; therefore, testing the blood or saliva for adrenal hormones should be done every 4 hours through a 24-hour period (cortisol test).

The Adrenal Type

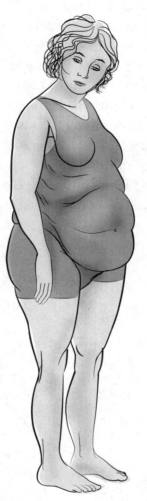

SAGGING, HANGING MIDSECTION WEIGHT WITH THIN ARMS AND LEGS

A fat pad can develop in the lower-neck and upper-back area, called a "buffalo hump."[2] I believe the reason the body creates this is to anchor the belly so you don't fall forward.

Fat accumulation in the face gives a round or "moon face" appearance.[3] The face also has redness because of weakened blood vessels.

Reddish purple striations (strips or bands resembling stretch marks) can appear on the stomach, thighs, buttocks, arms and breasts as well.

This type of individual generally has a large midsection with thin arms and legs. The reason is very interesting. The adrenal stress hormone cortisol breaks down leg muscle and turns it into sugar. This is a stress response by the body to supply quick energy; if you were being chased by a lion, you would need this energy. This sugar, if not completely burned up, will be converted to fat around the belly where the vital organs lie. The person's legs could eventually become thinner and weaker too, particularly at the knees. Cortisol will also take muscle from the buttocks, causing loss of tone in that area.

A common problem with the Adrenal type is the inability to fit into clothing, especially around the waist. Some people even wear elastic bands to hold the belly in, but this can constrict vital organs within the abdomen.

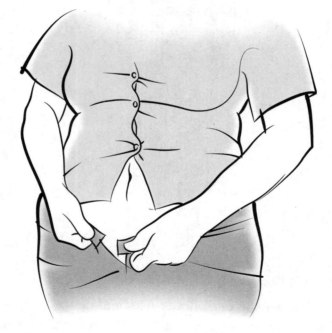

MIDSECTION WEIGHT

The pictures below show the changes from a normal body shape through the progressive stages of the Adrenal type.

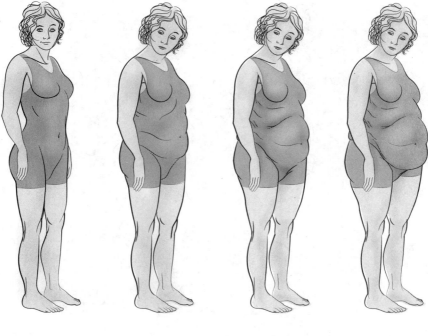

| NORMAL | STAGE 1 | STAGE 2 | STAGE 3 |

Cortisol can be very destructive on the body's proteins, especially bone tissue, leading to "thinning of the bones" (osteoporosis). It steals these proteins to use them as fuel, and during stress mode the body will go after any type of fuel, even your own body tissue. This might explain why some people have difficulty losing weight on high-protein diets.

High protein is supposed to trigger fat-burning hormones, but if the adrenals are releasing so much sugar from the tissues and even turning the muscles into sugar, these fat-burning hormones get blocked.

In this state, the body is trying to increase its survival by holding on to fat energy around the vital organs in the stomach area and the face. Of course, the body doesn't seem to care what the person will end up looking like. The face and eyes will become puffy, and a double chin and rounding of the face can develop.

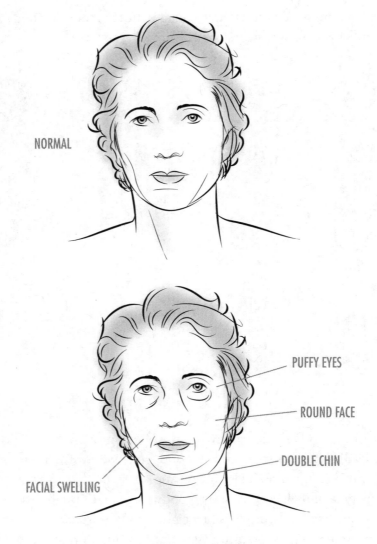

NORMAL

PUFFY EYES

ROUND FACE

DOUBLE CHIN

FACIAL SWELLING

SWOLLEN FACE AND EYES

In order to get into fat burning, there must be NO extra sugar or very limited sugar present in the blood. In the presence of sugar or refined carbohydrates, your body CANNOT and WILL NOT burn fat.[4] So, if the adrenals are constantly releasing sugar, how the heck are you supposed to lose weight?[5] In fact, sugar triggers the fat-storing hormone insulin, which will override all other fat-burning hormones and turn them off. The body will ALWAYS burn sugar in place of fat.

In women, adrenal hormone increases can result in a deeper voice, facial hair and male-pattern hair loss (receding hair line)—but other than that, the person is totally fine! I'm kidding. They can really mess with a woman's body.

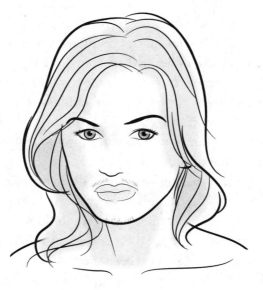

FACIAL HAIR

Acne can occur due to enlargement of the oil glands on the face, especially during women's periods. Atrophy (shrinkage) of the breasts can also be present. The above symptoms are due to an overabundance of male hormone production by the adrenals—androgens (*andro-* means "man").

Both the ovaries and adrenals produce estrogen and testosterone, which when out of balance can influence the oil glands and hair follicles. I have observed if a woman's right ovary is dysfunctional, the left side of her face (cheek) will develop more acne; and if the left ovary is out of balance, the right side of her face will develop more acne—there seems to be a crossover connection.

When excessive adrenal hormones are produced, the person has problems with the mineral calcium. In order to absorb calcium your blood needs to be a certain pH. This term *pH* refers to the acid/alkaline levels. The body has many fluids, which need to be either acid or alkaline. Overproduction of adrenal hormones can increase potassium loss, turning the person's blood pH on the side of too much alkalinity.[6] This prevents calcium from being directed to the bones and muscles, so one gets not only thinning of the bones but muscle cramps in the calves at night. Cramps in the calf muscles come from calcium, magnesium or potassium deficiencies. All three are adrenal problems. I think what's happening is instead of calcium going *into* the body it accumulates *on* the body tissues. I have observed these cases to have a buildup of tartar on their teeth, calcium on the eyes as early cataracts, on the bones as heel spurs, on the joints as arthritis, on the bursas (joint sacs) as bursitis, on the tendons as tendonitis, in the arteries as arteriosclerosis, deposits in the kidneys, and twitching under or on top of the left eyelid.

When the adrenals pump out excess hormones, high levels of calcium are lost through the urine, which is associated with osteoporosis.[7] Without this calcium, a person will have a difficult time getting to sleep, not to mention staying asleep. This is the cause of racing thoughts solving yesterday's problems at 2:00 a.m. when you should be sound asleep.

Leafy green vegetables are the best source of calcium—much better than milk. Pasteurized milk has been heated to a high temperature and, as a result, the calcium is much harder to absorb. A better source of dairy calcium would be plain yogurt or cheese. Yogurt and cheese are fermented and/or cultured products, and the friendly cultures and enzymes that are used reorganize amino acids (proteins), making a new food. These new proteins resemble plant proteins and are easier to digest and use by the body.

The adrenal hormones' timing mechanism (clock) controls circadian rhythms—waves of hormones that affect sleep and awake cycles. With adrenal problems everything is backwards; you are tired during the day, yet despite being exhausted you can't sleep through the night. The body just won't let you get into the deeper sleep cycles. Because the adrenals counter stress, their production of abnormally high amounts of stress hormones makes it impossible to attain the deep, restful sleep you need to properly rejuvenate the body for the coming day.[8]

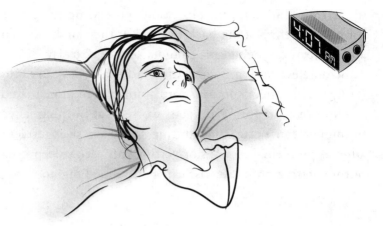

UNABLE TO GET RESTFUL SLEEP AT NIGHT

In the diagram below, you can see normal cortisol (adrenal hormone) levels. Notice that cortisol is supposed to be very minimal during sleep.

CIRCADIAN RHYTHM AND CORTISOL

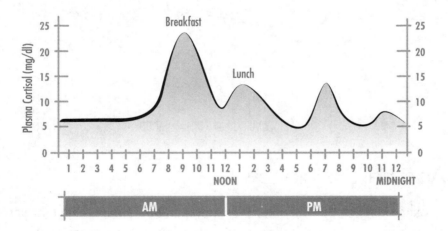

NORMAL ADRENAL HORMONE FLOWS

Certain adrenal hormones are responsible for making you feel awake mentally. Others are responsible for the sleep cycle.

Your body goes through four 90-minute cycles of sleep from superficial to deep. Just imagine trying to sleep while a lion was chasing you. You might be tired but your body would not be. Often a person will just wake up at 2:00–3:00 a.m. for no reason and end up lying there for an hour (or hours) before going back to sleep, if they are lucky. The worst thing about this is not being able to function the next day.

Because everything is backwards, Adrenal types can have bladder issues (leaky bladder, frequent urination) at night even more than during the day.

However, the problem gets worse. Fat-burning effects of certain hormones can occur only during the deep sleep cycles. But with an adrenal problem you are not getting into deep sleep cycles, so the fat-burning effects from exercise can get nullified due to poor sleep.

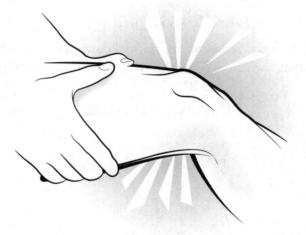

UNRESOLVING PAIN AND INFLAMMATION

Adrenal Deficiency

Exhausted adrenals can cause you to experience pain in different parts of the body because you are running out of anti-inflammatory hormones. If the "on-off switch" within the adrenals gets stuck, a person can go into a chronic stage in which pain and inflammation stay in the body for years. A person can also experience sore muscles that don't seem to recover after exercise. As this situation worsens, fibromyalgia develops, which is a condition of muscle pain throughout the entire body. What happens is there is an excess of inflammation throughout the body's muscles, tendons and connective tissues due to lack of the anti-inflammatory hormones normally produced by the adrenal glands. Having pain and inflammation and losing weight don't mix. The stress hormone triggered by the pain can block fat-burning hormones.

As far as muscle tissue is concerned, exercising with weights or doing high-pulse-rate exercise is not a good idea with this condition, since the extra stress overwhelms the adrenals. In chapter 17, you will learn more specifics for the Adrenal body type; adrenal exercise will involve walking and keeping your pulse rate no higher than 130 beats per minute.

Adrenal exhaustion will also cause overall body exhaustion with an inability to get restful sleep at night. Consequently, the Adrenal type of individual is usually fatigued, dragging their body around during the day, half awake.

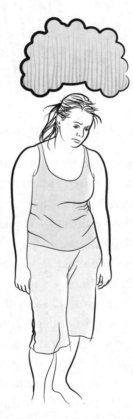

FATIGUED AND DRAGGING THE BODY AROUND

With weak adrenals, the person is more awake in the middle of the night than during the day. They can't get out of bed, feel tired after lunch, feel tired in the early evening, and if they don't get to bed at a certain time, then they can't go to sleep. If the Adrenal type has a sedentary job, they will have a wave of sleepiness right around 2:30–3:00 p.m. Due to a lack of quality sleep, midafternoon naps are desperately needed.

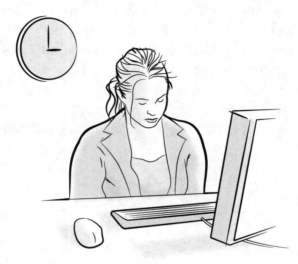

CAN'T STAY AWAKE MIDAFTERNOON

Typically, an individual with burnt-out adrenals has darkened circles under their eyes as well as a very tired appearance. They feel tired, drained and have brain fog. The brain fatigue can greatly affect concentration.

Adrenal types need coffee to wake up—strong Cuban coffee. Europeans use very small cups for coffee; Americans have humongous jugs of coffee. Caffeine—which is also in chocolate, sodas and tea—stimulates adrenal hormones and acts like an artificial energy booster, giving you mental alertness for one or two hours until it wears off. However, over time there are fewer highs and more lows. In college, I would drink pots of coffee at a time, trying to stay up at night and study. At that age most people can get away with it, but at 28 it caught up with me—stomach ulcers, insomnia, inflammation and severe fatigue. Over the years a person can feel depressed and very lethargic from this. Most people don't have depression; they just don't sleep!

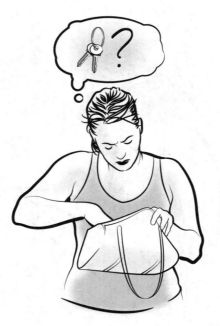

BRAIN FOG OR DULLNESS

Artificial sweeteners also aggravate these hormones. In my last book, I recommended Splenda as a substitute for sugar. In this book I am not recommending it because it could worsen the adrenals. I found a reference saying it could contribute to adrenal tumors in animals.

An interesting note about tea: Green tea, despite having some caffeine, has anti-caffeine properties and tends to not create the same jittery effect that drinking lots of coffee will. In some people it actually helps adrenal function.

If the adrenals do not work properly, this can affect oxygen levels, causing you to feel out of breath, particularly when the body is stressed, such as while climbing stairs.[9] The lower legs also will feel heavier, as if you were carrying around lead ankle weights, especially when you try to exercise on inclined surfaces.

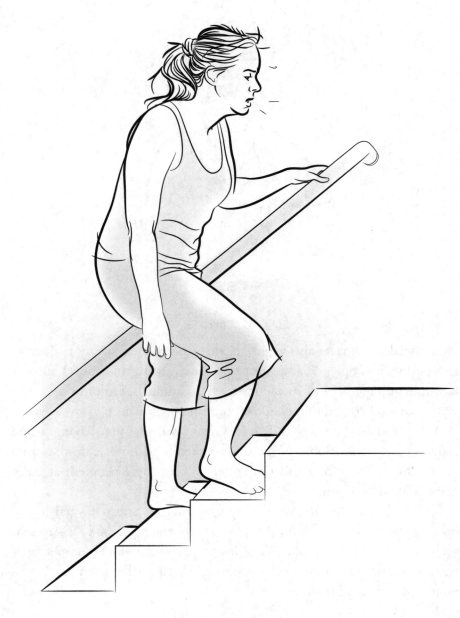

OUT OF BREATH WHILE CLIMBING

The adrenals have another function: controlling blood vessel contraction and relaxation, which affects blood pressure. Adrenal hormones constrict most blood vessels with the exception of two: the vessels in your lungs and the main artery around the heart (coronary). This is why a person with asthma needs a broncho (lung) steroid inhaler (which is adrenal hormones). If the adrenals can't relax the lungs, a constriction and tightening occurs preventing oxygen from entering. The coronary artery, which feeds oxygen to the heart muscle, is also controlled by the adrenal hormone adrenaline. If the adrenals are weak, the coronary artery can become constricted, especially under stress, preventing blood flow to the heart. This can give tightness in the chest or actual chest pains.

Are you beginning to see the importance of the adrenal glands?

Because the adrenals affect blood vessels, one can have abnormally constricted blood vessels in the inner ear, triggering ringing in the ears or even high blood pressure. High blood pressure could also stem from a calcium buildup in the arteries, since with adrenal problems a person tends to get arteriosclerosis (hardening of the arteries). Initially the top number (systolic) will increase before the bottom number (diastolic).[10]

There is a test called Ragland's in which you take a person's blood pressure lying down and then again standing up. Normally the top number (systolic) should rise 6 to 10 points when you stand up. However, with adrenal stress, the top number will either be lower than 6 points or higher than 10 points. (See illustration on the following page.)

If the person's test result is within normal range and they feel good after exercise, then a more intense workout would be indicated. If it is *not* within normal range and the person feels worse after exercise, then aerobic low-pulse-rate walking exercise would be recommended until the adrenals improve. You can find more on this in chapter 17.

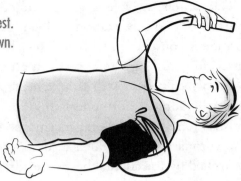

Lie down for 3 to 5 minutes' rest. Take blood pressure while lying down.

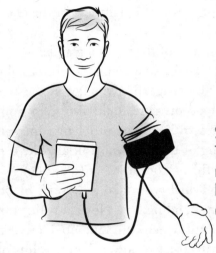

Stand and take blood pressure again. The top number (systolic) should normally rise 6 to 10 points. Having a higher or lower number could mean adrenal stress.

BLOOD PRESSURE TEST LYING, THEN STANDING

Stress responses to all aspects of life are the hallmark of the adrenals. People who have weak adrenals do not deal well with stress; the littlest things seem to irritate them rather easily. Excessive worry and anxiety are common with adrenal weakness due to the adrenaline stress response (fight or flight).

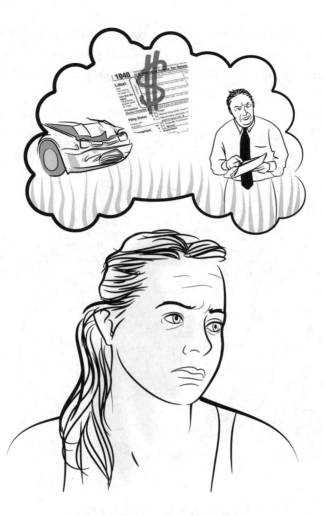

STRESS: EXCESSIVE WORRY AND ANXIETY ARE COMMON

When the adrenals decrease in function, the inability to handle life's stress increases. One patient of mine couldn't even sit through a movie that had any suspense; it would keep her up all night long. I had another patient who didn't have the patience to stand in line at the grocery store.

The adrenal-deficient case is usually worrying 24/7. This is very draining and leads to the need for stimulants—coffee, soda, tea and chocolate. These might give them an hour of clarity or feeling up, but the rest of the day is dull and lacking sharpness. This is the person who is half asleep and who is always visiting their local coffee shop.

Cravings for salt in the form of cheese, pretzels, nuts, popcorn or chips in the evening are common. People search the cupboards late at night for something crunchy and cheesy. This is because the adrenals regulate salts in the body.

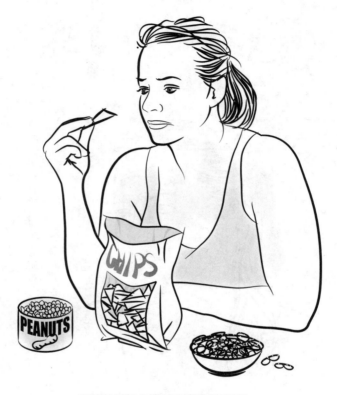

CRAVINGS FOR SALT OR CHEESE AT NIGHT

With salt and mineral imbalances, fluids can get out of balance, causing the individual to retain fluid (outside the cells) yet be dehydrated (inside the cells) at the same time.

Wherever sodium goes, water will accumulate. So when sodium gets lost through the urine, dehydration can occur. Often, drinking more water does not hydrate the person because there is too little sodium to balance it. In fact, I have found that people who drink the most water have the greatest dehydration.

FYI (for your information): Never consume table salt; use good quality sea salt. Sea salt has 84 minerals and table salt has only 2.

There is definitely a huge push for everyone to drink more water. Drinking more water so that you'll eat less usually won't satisfy you for more than 45 seconds. Instead it will make you feel bloated and cause you to get up several times during the night to use the bathroom, not to mention creating those little rings around your lower legs and ankles when you take off your socks at night.

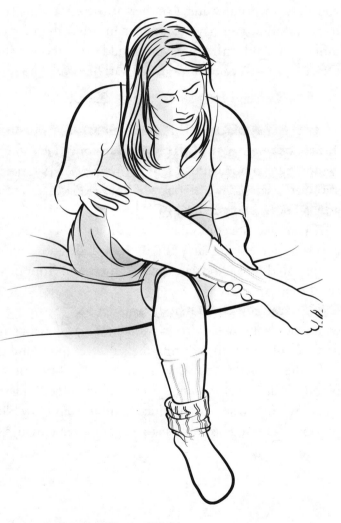

ANKLES SWELLING AT NIGHT

Many people make the mistake of drinking large quantities of water. I don't know who started the rumor that you need 8 to 10 glasses of water per day, or a gallon of ice-cold water—maybe the bottled-water companies. But if you drink too much of it, you can flush out minerals that are holding the water there in the first place, creating even more of an imbalance.

People use the same logic as they do for fat: If you are fat, you need to avoid fat calories; therefore, if your body is made mostly of water, then you need to drink water. Neither of these statements is true. In regard to fat calories, you have to understand that the hormones look at food differently. And with water, you should drink it only when you are thirsty. Don't ever force yourself to drink water—drink when you are thirsty!

FYI: Drinking water doesn't flush out fat.

A deficiency of adrenal hormones can also create cravings for chocolate. This is because some of the body's serotonin is produced by the adrenal glands. Serotonin creates a sense of well-being or comfort, and chocolate stimulates serotonin. People who crave chocolate are really craving the adrenal hormone serotonin.

If you take the combination of salt and chocolate, you get chocolate-covered pretzels. In fact, this is how I diagnose adrenal problems—I simply hold up a chocolate-covered pretzel in front of a person's face and see if they go for it.

The adrenals affect blood sugar levels.[11] So, poor adrenal function could cause the person to experience sugar cravings in addition to salt and chocolate cravings during the late afternoons and evenings.

In the following chart, you can see the different symptoms of high blood sugar and low blood sugar. High blood sugar (such as after a Thanksgiving meal) can produce brain fog, and low blood sugar can also produce brain fog, as well as anxiety and even cravings for sweets.

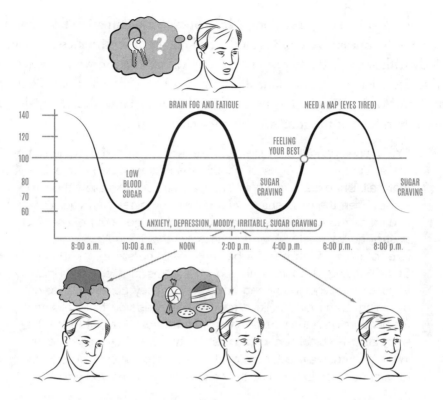

Your body will tell you what deficiency you have, based on what you crave. If you crave cheese or salt, this could mean you are low in sodium and your adrenal hormones are too low. If you crave grapefruit or melon, it could mean you're low in potassium and your adrenal hormones are too high. Craving licorice could indicate you are deficient in another adrenal hormone. The program I'm about to recommend will assist in giving the body what it needs so that you don't crave the wrong foods.

> FYI: Children who eat dirt or clay, or women who chew on ice during pregnancy, could be deficient in iron. (I would recommend eating beets instead of dirt.) Craving ice cream or cheese could also mean you are low in calcium, which indicates an adrenal problem.

Since the adrenal glands affect the immune system to a large degree, weakened adrenals can also cause increased susceptibility to viruses. Adrenal hormones suppress immune responses—such as inflammation, and itching of hives from excess histamine—as well as infections, viruses, etc. This is why when someone takes a steroid like prednisone—which is an adrenal hormone—the allergic reaction, asthma or even inflammation from poison ivy can disappear.[12] Allergies, asthma and chemical sensitivities occur in a body with weakened adrenals. This is the reason a person who experiences a severe allergy reaction (anaphylactic shock) needs what is called an EpiPen. An EpiPen is epinephrine (also known as adrenaline), which is a main hormone of the adrenals, in an injectable form.

> FYI: Viruses cannot be killed because they are not alive in the first place. Viruses are pieces of genetic material wrapped in a sac— that's all. But once inside your body, a weak cell can allow them to enter. When the virus enters your cell, it combines with your DNA and starts replicating. It's like a copy machine gone out of control, destroying your cells. A virus is so small that it would compare in size to a ping-pong ball if a bacteria were the size of the Empire State Building. It could fit through the pores of a porcelain dish. Viruses enter your body and never leave. They go into remission or hiding. Don't ever believe anyone who tells you to take some medication to kill the virus—it won't. Viruses can travel through the body into the spinal cord or brain and stay there. They are like seeds in the ground, waiting for the right environment. They wait for your resistance to be lowered so they can kick you when you are weak.
>
> The best defense against viruses, especially the flu, is to keep your resistance high by ensuring your adrenals are strong.

When the immune system goes crazy and starts to attack your own cells— autoimmune (self-attack)—the adrenal hormones are not doing their job. Normally, adrenal hormones are supposed to suppress immune cells. When this suppress function is broken, the immune system can go out of control.

The adrenals can overwork and underwork. Depending on the state they are in, you will experience different symptoms. I have frequently observed that a person will start with their adrenals in overdrive due to stress, then burn them out into an underworking adrenal situation. But it's not always that cut and dried, as a person might have a combination of symptoms. The eating and exercising program is designed to help normalize either overworking or underworking adrenals. Due to the destructive nature of the adrenals on your muscles, you may want to add a bit more protein with each meal. We'll cover more on this later when we get to tweaking your basic eating plan.

Causes of the Adrenal Body Type

There are several things that worsen or burn out the adrenal glands. The biggest of these is taking adrenal hormones; this could be in the form of prednisone or steroids (same thing). When you bypass the body and give it straight hormones, the adrenals don't have to produce their own. As a side effect this severely weakens the adrenals. I'm not recommending avoiding steroids if your doctor has advised them. I had a patient who was a swimsuit model; she developed a heel spur and received a steroid injection for pain. Four years later she developed a huge midsection with lots of stubborn weight. Steroids tend to make you put on weight by affecting the adrenals.

The second cause of adrenal problems comes from taking too much synthetic ascorbic acid (known as vitamin C). In nature, vitamin C comes in a whole-complex form, consisting of ascorbic acid, vitamin P factors (bioflavonoids), vitamin K and J factors, organic copper and the enzyme tyrosinase. The ascorbic acid antioxidant element is only one part. Taking this one part in huge doses can severely aggravate the adrenals, since the adrenal glands are a storage system for vitamin C. Man-made vitamin C (ascorbic acid) is often produced from cornstarch and sulfuric acid. You could even feel good taking these synthetics for a while, because they act as a stimulant. However, I've had patients take grams (1 gram is 1,000 milligrams) of the stuff and end up with adrenal problems down the road. Always take vitamin C in its whole form from food. In its whole form you rarely see the ascorbic acid part over 100 milligrams.

The third cause of weak adrenals is overwhelming stress to the body. Years of not sleeping, living with stressful people, a stressful environment, experiencing the loss of a loved one, going through a divorce, etc., can drain the adrenal glands.

The fourth cause of trouble with the adrenal glands is infection, especially from fungus, unfriendly yeast and viruses. The adrenals get a major amount of blood flow because they are above the kidneys. These microbes travel through the blood and get trapped in the adrenals and create problems later in life.

The fifth source of adrenal problems stems from a combination of taking stimulants and having nutritional deficiencies. Stimulants include caffeine, appetite suppressors, sugar, nicotine, synthetic vitamins, herbal stimulants (ma huang) and drugs. These items deplete vitamins (mainly B vitamins) and minerals (particularly potassium and calcium). Add in poor eating habits and lots of refined sugars and grains and you can end up with exhausted adrenals.

If the adrenal gland is involved, I recommend the adrenal nutritional support shown in the Resources section at the back of this book.

The following are symptoms the Adrenal type can experience from poorly working adrenal glands.

Adrenal Type Symptoms

- Pendulous abdomen (sagging and hanging)
- Midsection weight
- Buffalo hump (fat pad) at the upper-back, lower-neck area
- Thinner legs and arms
- Weakness
- Fatigue
- Lethargy
- Depression
- Sleepiness
- Insomnia
- Difficulty getting out of bed in the morning
- Need for midafternoon naps
- Nervousness
- Anxiety (worry); frequent feelings of stress
- Can't tolerate stress
- Thinning skin
- Acne or poor skin
- May have white or discolored patches on skin
- Reddish purple stretch marks on the stomach, thighs, buttocks, arms and breasts

- Red cheeks
- Round or moon face
- Puffy face and eyes
- Dark circles around eyes
- Double chin
- Facial hair
- Full eyebrows
- Receding hairline
- Deeper voice
- Sparse hair on forearms and lower legs
- Atrophy of breasts
- Tightness in chest, or chest pains
- High blood pressure
- Lax ligaments—weak ankles and knees
- Weak or brittle bones (due to a loss of calcium and protein)
- Difficulty absorbing calcium
- Needs coffee to wake up
- Salt, cheese, chocolate and sugar cravings, late afternoon and evening
- Inflammation or pain in joints, back, neck
- Heel spurs
- Overreactive immune system—allergies, chemical sensitivities
- Autoimmune conditions
- Fibromyalgia
- Asthma
- Increased susceptibility to viruses
- Dehydrated (intracellular) despite amount of water drunk
- Fluid retention in between cells
- Pitting edema (especially in ankles)
- Gets out of breath when climbing stairs
- Legs feel heavy, especially when exercising
- Moodiness and irritability
- Brain fog or dullness
- Ringing in ears
- Low sex drive

6

The Ovary Type

The Ovaries

The ovaries produce three hormones responsible for controlling the menstrual cycle. They release eggs every month and are in charge of making the environment suitable for the eggs' growth. One of these hormones is estrogen. It creates the fat layer around a female body, specifically around the ovaries—hips, buttocks and lower abdomen.

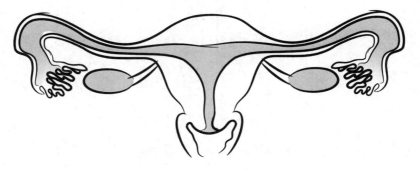

THE OVARIES

The Ovary Type

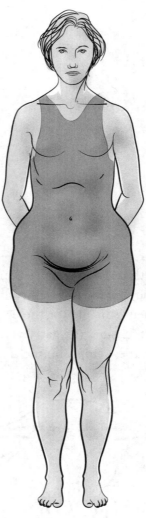

LOWER BODY WEIGHT—"SADDLEBAGS"

The following is a description of what happens when the ovaries don't function properly.

When ovaries become dysfunctional, they can produce an excess of estrogen, which causes more fat. I have observed that this fat is deposited on "saddlebag" thighs, the lower stomach and the buttocks. The lower-stomach fat usually shows up just below the bellybutton as a bulge.

Fat cells, by the way, also produce estrogen.

Problems that can be caused by the ovaries include PMS (premenstrual syndrome), cravings at certain times of the month, bloating at certain times of the month, extra painful cramps and excessive menstrual bleeding, as well as depression during the menstrual cycle. Apart from that, there is no problem at all!

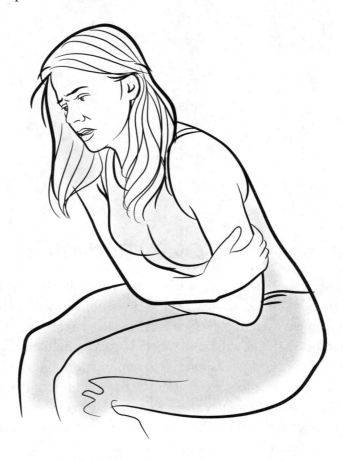

EXTRA PAINFUL CRAMPS

Many times a person with an Ovary body type experiences pain on either side of their lower-back area. Pain can also be in one of the knees, as the pain is being referred from one of the ovaries.

The pictures on the following page show the changes from a normal body shape through the progressive stages of the Ovary type.

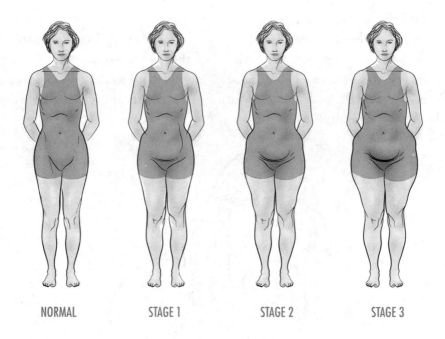

| NORMAL | STAGE 1 | STAGE 2 | STAGE 3 |

Causes of the Ovary Body Type

Ovaries are very sensitive to environmental hormones. Environmental hormones are those that come from birth-control pills, hormone replacement therapy (HRT) and other external supplies of hormones that enter the body. Growth hormones fed to beef, poultry and farm-raised fish are in this category. Chemicals that mimic hormones, such as pesticides and DDT, also affect the ovaries, uterus and breasts. Because the ovaries produce estrogen, when these external estrogens not produced by the body enter the system, the ovaries' own production becomes disrupted.

This can create one of two situations:

- The ovaries increase their production of estrogen, creating more fat deposits around the hips, thighs and lower stomach.

- The ovaries shut down their production of estrogen. When this happens, a part of the brain has to overcompensate and increase its hormone messages for the ovaries to produce more hormones. This is similar to a boss finding an employee not doing his job; he might then begin to put pressure on this individual to get back to work!

This second scenario is what can cause ovarian cysts and other growths. These cysts can make the affected ovary produce even more estrogen, resulting in additional fat around your thighs and hips. Pesticides on our foods can also act like estrogen and cause cysts, fibroids (fibrous growths) and tumors on the ovaries and uterus. They can create the same effect as environmental estrogens.

When a woman produces extra estrogen, the thyroid can get blocked. Anytime estrogen increases, as in pregnancy, the thyroid hormones are inhibited. The person might go to the doctor and have her thyroid checked, yet it isn't bad enough to show as being abnormal. A good endocrinologist will assess the entire endocrine system, including ovarian function.

It only takes very small amounts of estrogen and chemicals to create these effects; but by cleaning from the diet things that mimic estrogen, one can assist in bringing these hormones and glands back into a normal balance. For the Ovary type it is important to consume organic, hormone-free foods as much as possible.

The Menopause Backup Organ

During menopause the ovaries shut down. When this occurs the adrenal glands kick in and begin producing hormones similar to those the ovaries once produced, only in smaller quantities because the woman will not be giving birth. This fact is rarely known by the layperson. If the adrenal glands are weak or sluggish during menopause, they cannot act as the ovaries' backup organ and a person will usually start to have problems such as weight gain, hot flashes, night sweats and vaginal dryness.

A small part of the brain controls the ovaries. It is located right next to the temperature control center that affects perspiration, heart rate and sweating. When the ovaries shut down during menopause, if the adrenals cannot act as the backup the way they're supposed to, stress is placed on the controlling part of the brain. The lack of return communication from the adrenals to the brain creates stress in the perspiration center, causing a flush of heat and sweating. It could be likened to talking to or asking a question of your spouse while he or she is not responding to you. Being ignored would eventually upset you. In a similar way, your body reacts in the form of stress at the temperature center in the brain, which creates a flood of heat at any time of the day or night. That is what hot flashes are. Someone's trying to talk, but no one is listening.

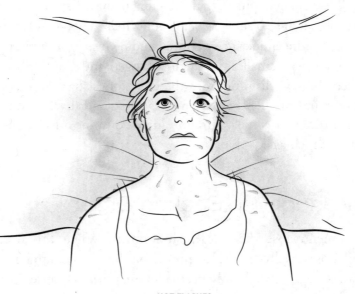

HOT FLASHES

The reason why HRT often helps with hot flashes is because it gives the brain a return message—the answer it is waiting for—thus calming everything down. It's an artificial reply, but it completes the circuit and turns off the heat. The only problem with this situation is some slight minor adverse complications seven years down the road—such as *strokes, heart disease, cancer* and *tumors of the liver*. Apart from that, it's totally safe!

I've observed that before age 52 the person might have a thinner waist with an Ovary body shape; then after age 52 she starts looking like an Adrenal shape (belly fat). This is because the adrenal gland is the backup to the ovaries.

The following are symptoms the Ovary type can experience from improperly working ovaries.

Ovary Type Symptoms

- Weight gain in hips, thighs and buttocks, with a lower-stomach bulge
- History of PMS
- Weight gain or bloating around that time of the month
- Ovarian cysts
- Cyclic fatigue
- Cyclic brain fog
- Cyclic pain in the lower back or hips
- Cyclic pain in the knee
- Cyclic lack of libido
- Infertility
- Hot flashes
- Night sweats
- Vaginal dryness
- Cyclic acne
- Cyclic mood swings
- Extra painful cramps
- Excessive menstrual bleeding
- Cyclic constipation
- Cyclic thinning of the hair
- Depression during menstrual cycle
- Cravings at certain times of the month

7

The Thyroid Type

The Thyroid Gland

Located in the lower part of the neck, and approximately 2½ inches wide, the thyroid gland regulates the rate at which the body burns food and controls the production of certain body tissues such as nails and hair. The thyroid gland also regulates body temperature, breakdown of carbohydrates, mental clarity and well-being, energy levels, and even vitamin absorption. Cholesterol levels, hair texture, nail strength, suppleness or dryness of the skin, and sex drive are all directly influenced by the thyroid.

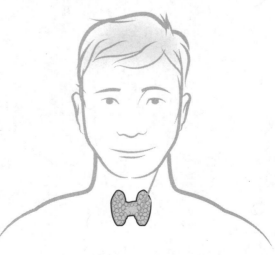

THE THYROID GLAND

The thyroid gland releases a combination of several different hormones. Their names aren't as important as their purpose—to speed up the metabolism of the body.

Metabolism refers to the rate or speed at which, or the degree to which, the body breaks down food and changes it into living tissue and energy. *Metabolism* also has a subdefinition, "the releasing of energy (burning of fat) from fat cells." And your metabolism is controlled by hormones.

The Thyroid Type

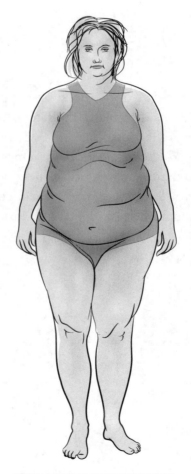

EXCESS FAT MORE EVENLY DISTRIBUTED

The Sluggish Thyroid

The first major consequence of a sluggish thyroid is a slow metabolism. Everything is slower. Brain processes can be suppressed, triggering depression, lethargy and a general apathetic feeling.

A loss of libido (sex drive) can occur with a slow thyroid. It could also cause a complete loss of the menstrual cycle.

Another manifestation is a feeling of being tired all the time, despite sleeping for long hours. This is chronic fatigue. Its distinct feature is feeling more awake in the morning but ready for bed at 8:00 p.m. The thyroid also controls the oil glands and blood flow to the skin. A sluggish thyroid can mean dry skin and dry, brittle hair. With a thyroid problem, a person could attempt to curl her hair and not be able to maintain the curl. She might even lose the outer third of her eyebrows.

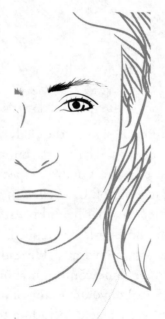

LOSS OF THE OUTER EYEBROWS

Since the thyroid gland controls metabolism, in a non-optimum state it begins to drive body temperature to well below normal, causing cold hands and feet. Sufferers need to wear extra clothing, even in moderate climates. Some people have to wear socks to bed. What's interesting is I've never met a person with cold feet who didn't have a spouse with warm feet—I guess opposites attract.

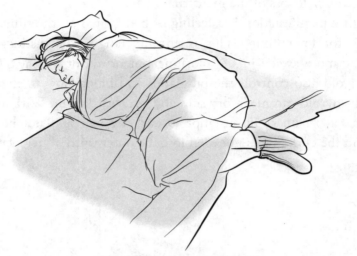

NEEDS TO WEAR SOCKS TO BED AT NIGHT

Because everything is slower, the body will demand quick energy, as in carbohydrate cravings. The most common cravings I have observed with the Thyroid type are starches, especially bread, and in particular sourdough bread just out of the oven with some butter.

I had this guy tell me that he didn't eat carbohydrates. I said, "Okay, what did you eat for breakfast?" He replied, "Apple pie from McDonald's." I told him, "That is carbohydrate." He said, "No it's not; it's apples."

There seems to be some confusion about what a carbohydrate is, so let me define it. A carbohydrate is any of a group of substances made of carbon, hydrogen and oxygen, including the sugars and starches. There are several types of carbohydrates: grains, vegetables, fruits and sugars. Unrefined carbohydrates provide vitamins and minerals as well as fiber, whereas refined grains have little nutrient value. Vegetable starches such as potatoes, yams, corn, french fries and hash browns are easily converted to fat, and some of the sweeter fruits have a greater effect on insulin.

The carbohydrates we are primarily concerned about are those that have been refined. Breads, pasta, cereals, crackers, pancakes, waffles, donuts, cakes, muffins, rice cakes, cookies, candy, chocolate, juice, alcohol, wine, beer and ice cream are all refined carbohydrates. And Thyroid types can crave any of these.

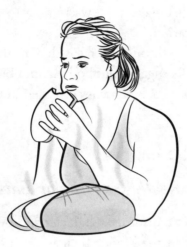

CRAVINGS FOR BREAD

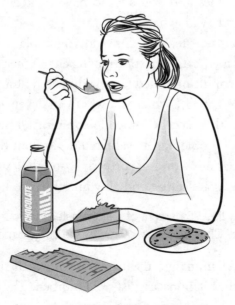

CRAVINGS FOR SUGARY CARBOHYDRATES

Have you ever eaten something that you knew you shouldn't have—at least once in your life? What have you normally said to justify it? "I deserve it." "I'll work out twice as hard tomorrow." "You have to die from something; might as well enjoy yourself." "If I eat it up, it won't be in the house to tempt me." "It doesn't count if no one sees me." "It's a holiday." "They wouldn't make it if it wasn't okay to eat"—or, my favorite, "Everything in moderation."

The main problem with burning fat is this: in the presence of refined carbohydrates (especially sugar), your body cannot burn fat. I'm sorry! And to top it off, the excess carbohydrate is converted into fat and cholesterol.[1]

High Cholesterol

Are You Sure It's Really Genetics or Eating Fatty Foods?

There are rare genetic disorders characterized by an accumulation of large quantities of fat in the blood. If they're rare, how do you explain the millions of people who have high cholesterol? Some people will even tell you it's bad genes and you should have picked your parents more wisely. Good luck! And what about eating fat—does that cause high cholesterol? If that is true, then how do you explain why a person still needs cholesterol medication despite having cut all the fat out of their diet? There is another condition called familial hypercholesterolemia (excessive cholesterol in the blood), which shows up in seven out of a thousand people. So, rather than accept someone's opinion on whether you have a genetic cholesterol problem, get evaluated to find out the facts. The point is, if your thyroid is not working correctly, your cholesterol could be high in spite of what you are eating and all your efforts to keep it low.

> Did you know that 75 percent of the cholesterol in your body is made by your body? Cholesterol is required by the body to make hormones.

The need for vitamins greatly increases with a thyroid weakness. The weakness means the vitamins are just not absorbed. The body dumps them through the urine—expensive urine because these vitamins are wasted. Such people are usually taking vitamin supplements and not feeling any different.

By the way, what was the first vitamin that was ever discovered? Was it C? No. How about D? No. The answer is A. Then came B, then C, then D and E.

The body-fat pattern resulting from a sluggish thyroid is an overall fat distribution. The pictures below show the changes from a normal body shape through the progressive stages of the Thyroid type.

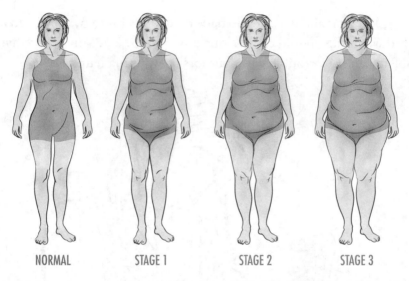

NORMAL   STAGE 1   STAGE 2   STAGE 3

As a side note, a person with a true sluggish thyroid problem is not solely retaining fat. They have a great deal of waste-like-fluid weight that contributes to the appearance of having an overall excess weight problem. As mentioned previously, this condition is called myxedema and is the result of a thyroid that is not working to full capacity.

Many people think they have attention deficit disorder (ADD) when in fact they may have a weak thyroid. Have you ever known people who walked into a room and forgot why? Have you ever talked to someone you could tell was a bit checked out? This type of lethargy can be attributed to poor thyroid function. And without really spending the time to evaluate and find the true cause, a person could be put on Ritalin by mistake.

I really think the problem with our healthcare system narrows down to incomplete evaluation. If you have pain, you are given a pill; high blood pressure—pill; high cholesterol—pill; ADD—pill. This is what I call duct-tape therapy. There is very little discovery of underlying causes to these problems. If it were HEALTHcare it would work; but it's disease care. There's hardly any prevention or food therapy. Even worse is the lazy diagnosis—you know, "You're getting older now and you have to accept the fact that these things come with age." Or, "It's your genetics; you have the fat gene." Or, "You're African American and at risk for _____ , so take these pills the rest of your life." Everything is heavy on treatment but very light on prevention or evaluation to find the real cause.

The skin, hair and nails are all made up of body protein, which becomes altered when the thyroid can no longer do its job. A person with a thyroid problem can have trouble with hair loss or thinning hair.

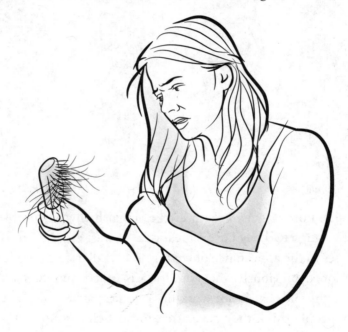

HAIR LOSS OR THINNING HAIR

Sagging skin under the arms, chin or midsection can occur because the body protein that holds the skin firm is breaking down faster than it is building up. Have you ever met someone with these symptoms—a friend, neighbor, relative or co-worker?

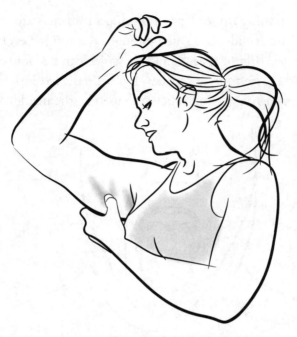

LOOSE SKIN UNDER UPPER ARMS

Your nails especially are made from protein, and because the person's body protein is breaking down faster than it can be built up, the fingernails can become brittle with prominent vertical (up-and-down) ridges.

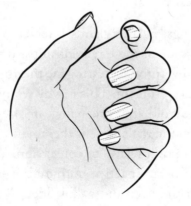

VERTICAL RIDGES ON THE NAILS

A poorly functioning thyroid gland produces puffiness around the eyes and sagging of the eyelids. If it's bad enough, the tongue even thickens, causing a slight slurring of speech, and the voice can become deeper and rougher in sound. The tongue can develop little dished indentations on the sides; it is getting bigger and is being shaped by the inside of the teeth.

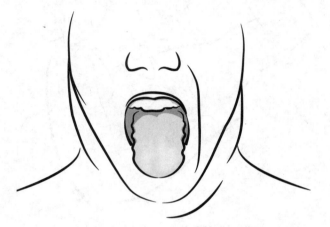

INDENTATIONS ON SIDES OF TONGUE

The Thyroid Problem Is Usually Secondary

To complicate things, all the glands interact with one another, and we earlier looked at some of these relationships. In regard to the thyroid gland, if the ovaries overproduce estrogen, the thyroid will decrease in function as a secondary problem. This is why women notice weight gain and even a sluggish thyroid after pregnancy, or after taking birth-control pills or being on hormone replacement therapy.

Another important point relates to conversion. Your thyroid hormone in the form called T4 is an inactive hormone. It is changed to T3, the active form, through the liver and gallbladder. Without a healthy liver and gallbladder, it doesn't matter if you have additional T4 because your body will not allow it to work. Since 80 percent of thyroid function occurs through the liver, unless the liver is working well a good portion of thyroid function will be missing.

There are actually three reasons why people may be taking thyroid hormones yet never see any changes with energy or weight loss: (1) The estrogen is so dominant that the thyroid function is being impaired. (2) The gallbladder or liver is damaged; thus very little conversion of thyroid hormone is taking place. And (3), if your adrenals become dysfunctional, an autoimmune condition with your thyroid can develop; this is called Hashimoto's or Graves' disease. This is why there is always a stress event just before these conditions start.

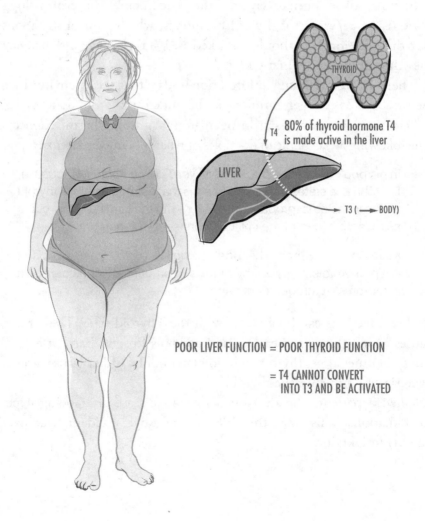

THYROID

T4 80% of thyroid hormone T4 is made active in the liver

LIVER

T3 (——→ BODY)

POOR LIVER FUNCTION = POOR THYROID FUNCTION

= T4 CANNOT CONVERT INTO T3 AND BE ACTIVATED

People frequently ask me what to do to fix their thyroid. Well, first of all ask yourself which symptoms are the most evident: Do you have mostly bloating or digestive issues? Do you have mostly high-estrogen symptoms? Or did you experience a stress event just before your thyroid became dysfunctional? These questions will help you narrow the problem down to the most likely source. Then, in the Resources section at the back of this book, you can look into nutritional support that can assist greatly.

Causes of the Thyroid Body Type

Some medical journals say that the fundamental cause of a sluggish thyroid is a *deficiency* of thyroid hormones, which control metabolism. But the question that should be asked is, WHY is there a deficiency of these hormones in the first place?

There is accumulating information today that toxic environmental factors, such as estrogen mimics, can be linked to thyroid deficiencies.

Scientists who study poisons in the environment are finding this connection. The following are a couple of examples of what is being discovered.

> In his book *What Your Doctor May Not Tell You about Menopause*, Dr. John Lee states: "My hypothesis is that estrogen inhibits thyroid action in the cells, probably interfering with the binding of thyroid to its receptor" [part of the cell that connects with hormones].[2]

> Mary Shomon writes in her book *Living Well with Hypothyroidism*: "Hypothyroidism [low thyroid] is sometimes considered a symptom of estrogen dominance."[3]

Past infections can be a factor with the Thyroid type. The virus that causes Mono (kissing disease), also known as Epstein-Barr virus (EBV), can sometimes affect thyroid function later in life. Other viruses and even bacteria can influence the thyroid.

I had a patient who developed thyroid disease after being exposed to radiation. This was the 1986 Chernobyl accident (radioactive fallout) in Ukraine.

Your own ovaries could be causing your thyroid problem (unless you're a man, of course). A cyst or fibroid on the ovary can produce excessive estrogen in the body. This includes polycystic ovarian syndrome (PCOS)—a condition where multiple small cysts form in the ovaries (*poly* means "many"), related to the ovary's failure to release an egg. PCOS can create facial hair, weight gain, insulin resistance and a disruption in the menstrual cycle. So, there could be primary ovarian problems causing a secondary thyroid problem. This could trigger thyroid symptoms, yet the true problem would be the ovaries.

> FYI: If you have PCOS, I would recommend avoiding all estrogen triggers—hormones in our food supply, soy products, and foods that have been sprayed with pesticides; consume organic produce as much as possible. One of my female patients always had a flare-up of cysts when she ate commercial ice cream, which contained extra hormones and chemicals.

Another activity that inhibits thyroid hormones is low-calorie diets. When you cut calories, your thyroid compensates by lowering the metabolic rate. However, people confuse cutting calories with intermittent fasting. Low-calorie diets create nutritional deficiencies, which result in cravings and hunger; whereas with intermittent fasting you are decreasing only the frequency of eating without restricting calories, and making sure that your meals are nutrient dense and satisfying. We will be looking at intermittent fasting in more detail in later chapters.

Estrogen

Estrogen inhibits thyroid function.

Some women develop thyroid problems after pregnancy due to the high levels of estrogen produced; and if a woman who has a thyroid weakness goes through pregnancy, her thyroid medication will usually need to be increased.

These statements raise two key questions: If estrogen inhibits thyroid function, then how are we being exposed to increased amounts of estrogen? And how much estrogen exposure does an average person get on a daily basis?

Estrogen is the number one hormone added to the feed of animals we consume. It is fed to cattle, turkeys, chickens and farm-raised fish. This hormone makes these animals grow faster and plumper. It is more costly, for example, to grow hormone-free chickens for 22 weeks than to grow hormone-fed chickens for only 6 weeks. I believe out of all the things that go into your body, commercial milk contains the highest amount of estrogen. Always drink organic milk, if you're going to drink it at all.

Most European countries do not use growth hormones on their animals, and some refuse to buy American hormone-fed meats. Could this be why Americans are fatter?

A common argument against this concept is that the hormone amounts given to animals are so small they have no effect upon the body. But there is far too much evidence available that supports the effects of estrogen. It takes very minute amounts of estrogen in the body to create effects.[4] And pesticides, insecticides, DDT and many other chemicals mimic estrogen in the body, adversely affecting the thyroid.

Another common argument is, if these chemicals are this damaging to our hormones, why doesn't the Environmental Protection Agency advise the public of the thyroid-chemical connection? The reason is that there is a long delay time between exposure and showing symptoms, which makes it hard to pinpoint the actual cause. It could take more than 30 years.

If you have a Thyroid body type, I highly recommend you reduce your dietary food exposure to estrogen by eliminating foods that contain growth hormones. It would also help to reduce the consumption of chemicals (pesticides, insecticides, DDT, etc.) that mimic this hormone, by either introducing organic foods into your diet or at least scrubbing your fruits and vegetables before eating them.

Red wine unfortunately has estrogen-like compounds. I would advise cutting back to no more than two bottles a night—I'm just kidding. You need to avoid all alcohol on this program. Come on, we need to give your liver a break! I know what you are saying—you drink it for health reasons, right?

Cruciferous Vegetables and Iodine

Cruciferous vegetables, which belong to the cabbage family, include kale, radishes, Brussels sprouts, cabbage, bok choy, etc.—you know, the foods that people normally never eat. Cruciferous vegetables are anti-iodine, meaning they tend to deplete iodine, which the thyroid needs in order to function.[5] When I say "tend to deplete iodine," I mean very slightly. You would have to eat ALL cruciferous and nothing else to create this effect. Most of the other foods you eat put the iodine right back, so I wouldn't be too concerned. But if you feel unsure about this and want to eat cruciferous vegetables, just take some extra iodine from sea kelp; then go ahead and receive the benefits of these vegetables, because they are also anti-estrogen foods. I believe their benefits far outweigh any liability.

I have created a product to help support healthy estrogen levels, called **Organic Cruciferous Superfood**. Not only does it contain organic cruciferous vegetables, but it also includes sea kelp (see Resources section).

If You Are Missing Your Gallbladder

If you are missing a gallbladder, we need to find it and stick it back under your liver . . . I am kidding again; it's probably gone for good. But interestingly, gallbladders do have a tendency to grow back, in some situations. Normally the gallbladder stores bile and concentrates it at 500 percent. As you eat, the bile gets released. Without a gallbladder, bile merely trickles down a tube (bile duct) from the liver directly into the small intestine. As a result, you get less bile and a much weaker concentration of bile. This can show up in incomplete fat digestion and vitamin A, D, E and K deficiencies, which relate to poor night vision, dry skin, and calcium metabolism problems as well as hormone problems.

If you have no gallbladder or you seem to have gallbladder symptoms, I recommend taking purified bile salts. See the Resources section for the Gallbladder Formula.

The following are symptoms the Thyroid type can experience from a poorly working thyroid gland.

Thyroid Type Symptoms

- Weakness
- Fatigue
- Lethargy
- Sleepiness
- Need for midafternoon naps
- Generalized weight gain
- Sagging skin under arms, chin or midsection
- Low/poor appetite
- Craving bread, pasta, chocolate, sweets
- High cholesterol
- Brittle nails with vertical ridges
- Hair stiff and dry
- Hair loss or thinning hair
- Dry skin
- Puffiness around eyes
- Sagging eyelids
- Outer eyebrows thinning or absent
- Slight rosiness or reddening of the face
- Poor short-term memory and focus
- Depression
- Apathetic (loss of hope)
- Difficulty making decisions
- Low body temperature
- Cold intolerance (need to put on a sweater or more covers while sleeping)
- Cold feet and/or hands
- Loss of libido
- Loss of menstrual cycle
- Indentations on sides of tongue
- Thickening of tongue
- Voice deeper and rougher in sound

8

The Liver Type

The Liver

The liver is the body's filtration system. It filters out microbes, drugs and dead cells from the body as an immune function. Every hormone, chemical, bacteria, virus, fungus and parasite is filtered through the liver. It is similar to an oil filter in your car. In addition, it acts as a digestive organ, breaking down fats, proteins, and even carbohydrates. It can also make sugar out of protein.

The liver is a major organ for detoxification; it works to break down the chemicals taken in from toxins on foods to which you are exposed daily. It uses sulfur to break down toxic chemicals into harmless ones. Eggs, cruciferous vegetables (e.g., broccoli, cabbage, Brussels sprouts, cauliflower and kale), raw garlic and onions are rich sources of sulfur.

Cruciferous vegetables have some unique properties, including being anti-estrogenic and anti-carcinogenic (anti-cancer causing); and since many hormone problems stem from excessive estrogen and toxins, it would be wise to eat as many of these vegetables as possible. In fact, they are the central food for a Liver type.

When the liver gets damaged over the years, toxins that are normally filtered out can recirculate through the body, re-exposing delicate glands to harmful compounds, triggering a toxic overload. Synthetic estrogen from growth hormones, medications, aspirin, birth-control pills and HRT (hormone replacement therapy) also causes huge side effects of damage to the liver.

The liver has over 500 known functions, and every fat-burning hormone works through the liver.

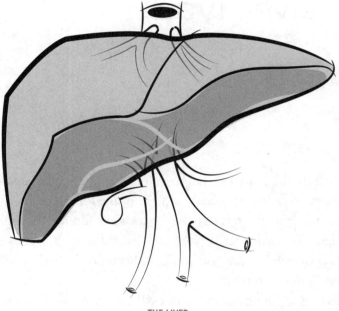

THE LIVER

The following is a description of what happens when the liver does not function properly.

When damaged, the liver causes a potbelly appearance. This protruding abdomen is not always fat; it could be fluid. If the liver is not functioning well it can leak fluid into the stomach area within the abdomen. This characteristic is called *ascites*, which comes from the Greek *askos*, meaning "bladder," "belly" or "wineskin" (animal skin used to hold wine). If you push the stomach from side to side, it looks and feels like a water balloon. An ultrasound is the best way to confirm fluid in the abdomen.

The Liver Type

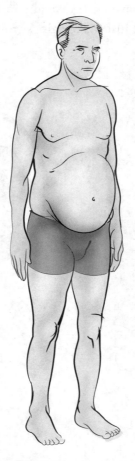

PROTRUDING STOMACH—POTBELLY

Have you ever seen the skinny guy with a potbelly on the beach wearing a Speedo? Sorry for the image. One female patient told me, "Yes, I think I've seen this person before . . . every night before I go to bed!" That is ascites—water weight in the abdomen. There is a sac inside the abdomen area that fills up as the improperly working liver leaks liquid. The fluid is leaking because the liver is not able to produce proteins—it's a low-protein situation that can't be fixed by just eating more protein. You can only improve this by eating high-quality proteins and lots of vegetables that take the stress off the liver and let it heal. This has also been called a "beer gut," which creates the same stomach because alcohol destroys the liver. If you happen to have excess weight in the midsection, a glass of wine or beer at night will just make things worse.

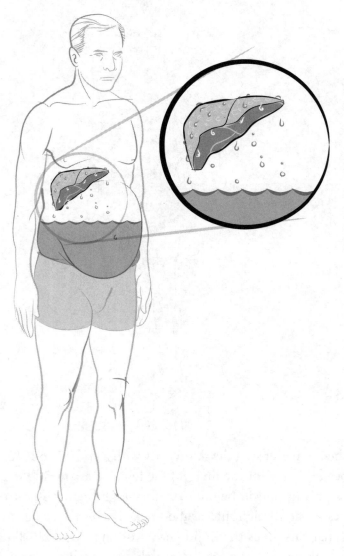

FLUID IN ABDOMEN—ASCITES

The pictures below show the changes from a normal body shape through the progressive stages of the Liver type.

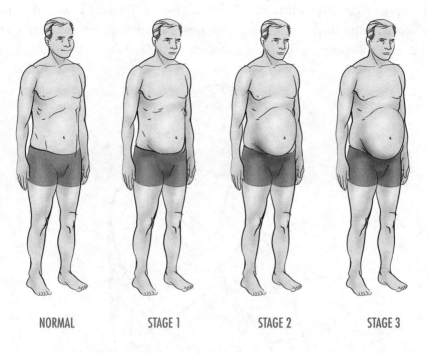

NORMAL   STAGE 1   STAGE 2   STAGE 3

Liver types usually have a dull pressure and fullness in the upper abdomen just under the right rib cage. Some of these people get tired for a while after each meal. When they lie on their left side at night, it becomes uncomfortable due to a swelling of the liver, which compresses the heart. Lying on the right side seems to be the most comfortable because the heart can rest on top of the liver. They are sensitive to a whole range of foods, especially fatty foods and refined grains, and must eliminate grains altogether or suffer the consequences of bloating, gas and indigestion.

There is a tight, almost arthritic-like feeling in the lower back, particularly in the morning. There is also a tightness or pain in the right shoulder or right side of the neck, which they will swear is an old injury, but treatments to the right shoulder never seem to resolve it long term. The reason is because the right shoulder is just the tip of the iceberg.

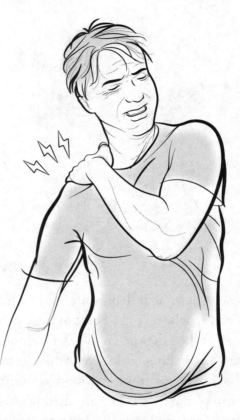

TIGHTNESS, PAIN AND STIFFNESS IN THE RIGHT SHOULDER OR NECK

The tongue has a deep split down the center and is often coated with a white film. The head frequently feels heavy and dull with aches in the forehead and neck area, and the person usually wakes up an hour before needing to get out of bed. In other words, the Liver type rarely gets the last part of sleep, resulting in inadequate sleep. The Adrenal type, on the other hand, sometimes gets up every 90 minutes or every two to three hours.

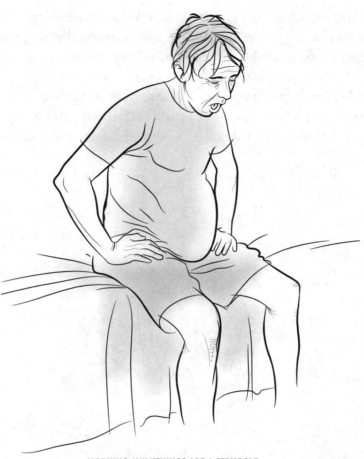

MORNING AWAKENINGS ARE A STRUGGLE

The morning is a struggle. This is because the liver can't hold blood sugar for a full seven hours; so morning grouchiness is actually coming from low blood sugar. When the person doesn't eat for a ten-hour span (from dinner to the next morning), the amount of sugar in the blood is excessively depressed, creating irritableness, moodiness, mentally depressed feelings and lethargy, most noticeable upon waking. Many Liver types become more pleasant to be around in the evening after several meals.

The urine is usually darker in the morning and becomes increasingly watery and clearer as the day progresses. Being similar to the oil filter in your car, the liver can get dirty.

The whites of the eyes can show a tint of yellow and can be very bloodshot in the morning as well. The eyelids may become itchy and swollen.

Arthritis and bad skin are also indicative of liver damage.[1] The finger joints, particularly in the morning, become stiff and slightly swollen. This worsens if refined grains were consumed the night before, since many Liver cases have difficulty with gluten (the protein part of grains). Wheat and other grain products seem to aggravate arthritis and cause joint pain and inflammation in various parts of the body (mid back, low back, lower neck, hands, right shoulder, ankles, and even in the knees).

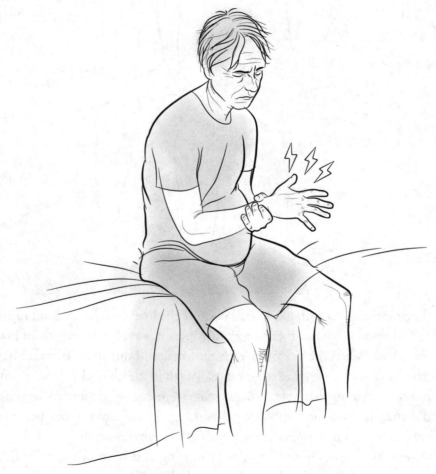

STIFF, SORE AND SWOLLEN FINGER JOINTS IN THE MORNING

When refined grains are avoided, the arthritis many times disappears. The body seems to misidentify the gluten in these grains as a microbe, creating an inappropriate immune response. The only grains that don't have gluten are rice, millet, spelt and oats. However, I'm recommending avoiding all grains on this diet.

Digestive problems are also a characteristic of the Liver type. This includes bloating, constipation and acid reflux.

Liver types will often crave the very foods that will destroy the liver—fatty foods, bacon, chips and deep-fried foods, especially from fast-food restaurants. When they are hungry, fried catfish, breaded onion rings or french fries look very appetizing. But after eating these foods, they will feel bloated, as their digestive systems are poor, and they'll usually start burping and belching after a high-fat meal.

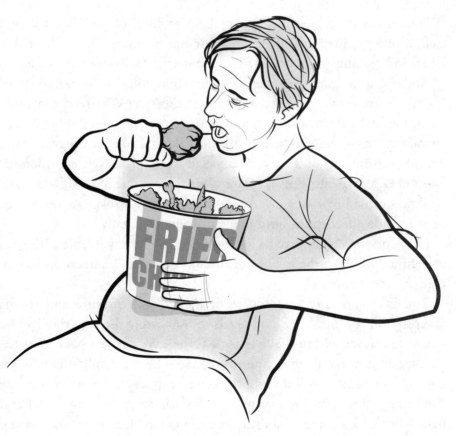

CRAVINGS FOR FATTY FOODS

If the liver is weakened, the person might get brown spots on the backs of their hands and throughout the body, called liver spots. Other skin issues that can occur are red dots, psoriasis, eczema, and even fungal growths on the scalp and toenails.

Itching is the most significant clinical symptom of severe liver cell damage.[2] The person seems to be always scratching something on their body; they experience itchiness especially at night. The itchiness usually occurs because the liver fluids are backing up into the blood.

With an advanced liver problem, the fingers occasionally look clubbed (blunted and squarish) and the nail beds appear whitened.[3] The nail bed should normally have a pinkish color.

As the liver becomes progressively more destroyed, the person's breath develops a distinct odor, musty and sweetish. If you ever visited a sick room in the hospital, you'd notice this smell.

Sometimes the bowel movements become light colored because of a lack of bile production. Bile is the substance produced by the liver that assists in breaking down fats. It's like the soap that dissolves the grease.

And because the liver has a main function of breaking down chemicals and environmental hormones, excessive estrogens can build up in the body. In major cases, a male body can start developing female characteristics—enlarged breasts, thinned skin, and even a higher voice. Atrophy (shrinkage) of the testes can occur from this as well. Another side effect of excessive estrogens is spider veins. This is due to the blood vessel weakness caused by estrogens. As you might know, strokes are one of the negative side effects from hormone replacement therapy.

I have personally observed a loss of memory in many people with poor liver function. Even the medical textbooks describe "brain confusion" as part of liver problems.[4]

The liver can also be a source of high blood pressure and edema (swelling) in the ankles.[5] Blood needs to flow freely through the liver, so any obstructions within the liver (scar tissue) will create a back pressure.

Excessive scar tissue can occur in a damaged liver, a condition known as cirrhosis. In order to call it cirrhosis, however, it has to be major scarring; if it's only minor scarring it can't be called cirrhosis. It is my belief that many people have some minor scarring, enough to block liver function and cause weight gain and fluid retention in the abdomen. There are situations whereby cirrhosis is reversible, provided the damaging triggers are removed and sufficient time is allowed for a return to normal liver structure.

The liver is definitely one organ that has the capacity to totally rejuvenate. It is constantly repairing itself, yet there is a point where it gets overwhelmed.

Causes of the Liver Body Type

A liver problem can originate from many different sources. One is constipation. If the bowels cannot eliminate, the liver will become backed up. The toxicity in the body will prevent weight loss. A woman with this situation came to see me, who had received one of the introductory offers in my email health tips inviting her to come in for a free consultation. When she showed up at the office, she was close to 400 pounds. She told me she had driven from Michigan to my clinic in Virginia for one consultation to help her lose weight. Then I found out she was having only one bowel movement per month! And she was more interested in weight loss. I explained that her bowels had to be handled before she could even think about losing weight. I never saw her again—her bowel problem wasn't a concern.

Another source is the consumption of refined sugars, which include hidden sugars such as juice and alcohol. The liver is the first line in the chain of organs that deal with sugar. When you eat lots of sugar, the liver is forced to handle it.[6] This creates major stress on the liver.

Sugar (as in cake, candy and other sweets) breaks down so fast it shocks the liver, making it weaker. On the other hand, vegetables break down so slowly you'll never have to worry about overeating them; the nutrition level is so high in vegetables that your body just won't let you eat too many. But if you take carbohydrates in their refined form—white sugar, alcohol, breads or even fruit juices—it's easy to overeat, since nutrition is low and the body won't tell you when to stop. Vitamin and mineral levels in food signal the brain and tell it when it is satisfied. Refined foods are stripped of their nutrition. The fiber in vegetables turns off the hunger switch as well.

What many people don't fully understand is that sugar, breads, pasta, cereals, crackers, pancakes, waffles, juice and soda are equally hard on the liver. All will be converted to either fat or cholesterol. The mixture of sugars with fats—in the form of ice cream, barbecue ribs and breaded meats—adds stress to the liver too.

Consuming excessive quantities of proteins and fats also puts damaging stress on the liver cells.

The liver produces substances to break down fats, but when it is deficient, an overload of fatty foods aggravates the liver. This shows up as tightness around the chest (just below the ribs), pain or tightness in the right-shoulder area, belching or burping, and bloating in the digestive system.

Cravings for fatty foods come from the body telling you it needs something. What? It needs the fat-soluble vitamins—A, D, E, K and certain B vitamins. If you listen to your body, it will explain what it needs. Sausage, meatloaf, bacon, overly cooked greasy roast beef, deep-fried onion rings, french fries, breaded meats, greasy barbecue ribs, are all hard on the liver and its associated gallbladder. Eating raw beets (grated over salad) or steamed beets (not canned) each day will make the Liver type feel very good. Beets thin the bile and are also great for constipation.

A further big cause of liver problems is toxic chemicals. This is another way in which estrogens from the environment, along with pesticides and insecticides like DDT, adversely affect the body. These substances become trapped in the liver and create altered function.

Viruses and fungi can destroy the liver, hepatitis being a common liver problem. When a person takes excessive antibiotics, he or she can end up with all sorts of fungi, unfriendly bacteria, yeast and candida. Candida is a yeast-like fungus that is normally in balance with other friendly microbes; but an overgrowth of candida, which spreads on the tongue and private parts, can occur after antibiotic use. If you have this situation, to replace the good bacteria consume more fermented foods: pickles, apple cider vinegar, kimchi and sauerkraut. It is not true that people with yeast need to avoid friendly yeast foods—just the opposite.

High-cholesterol drugs have been known to weaken the liver. Since many side effects from medications affect the liver, the liver is a common weak link in a large percentage of the population.

Liver damage could be brought about through nutritional deficiencies, especially the B vitamins. I'm not recommending going out and taking some synthetic vitamins, as they can create other problems. I would recommend avoiding refined foods, which deplete B vitamins. Breads, pasta, cereals and flour products are usually enriched with B vitamins because during the refining process B vitamins are destroyed. However, just spraying some synthetic vitamins doesn't fix this problem. Consuming refined-grain products and refined sugar depletes the body primarily of B vitamins and potassium. A very good source of the B vitamins is nutritional yeast, from either the health food store or Amazon.com. One teaspoon per day would be wise. Make sure you don't confuse this with brewer's yeast or baker's yeast; get the non-fortified nutritional yeast.

And by the way, synthetic B vitamins are made from coal tar, not food. Always consume vitamins from food. The foods must be listed on the label. If you see 50 milligrams of B_1, 50 milligrams of B_6, etc., then you can be pretty sure they are synthetic. Food concentrates come in smaller and different quantities, such as 3.4 milligrams or 32.4 milligrams.

Consuming processed prepared foods high in MSG (monosodium glutamate) damages the liver. This is a way to take massive quantities of sodium without tasting the saltiness of it. The next day the hands get swollen and the ankles have edema lines when you take off your socks, not to mention that blood pressure increases.

Many people avoid salt or sodium if they have high blood pressure. Why not increase the opposing mineral, potassium? In this program, you will be consuming large quantities of potassium-rich foods. High-potassium, low-sodium foods would be all the leafy greens, kidney beans, avocados, honeydew melon and sea kelp.

Testing for Liver Damage

Liver damage often will not show up on blood tests; even significant damage may show normal findings on liver tests.[7] The liver is rugged and takes lots of abuse, so there can be considerable damage before any symptoms are present. I had one patient who was an alcoholic from age 14 through 42. He has been dry for ten years, but it's amazing he's not dead.

The most accurate way to determine liver damage is through a biopsy; of course, that's a bit invasive. Ultrasound of the abdomen can tell if the person is carrying fluid (ascites), but other tests might not tell the full story. Normal liver enzymes are not a good indicator of the absence of liver damage. Many people have normal levels yet have advanced liver disease.

Creating a Healthy Liver

Because all fat-burning hormones create their effects through the liver, having a healthy liver is the most important first step in weight loss. Without a healthy liver, fat burning will be next to impossible.

The best foods for the liver are raw cruciferous vegetables and small amounts of lean proteins (raw nuts, fish, etc.). Since a damaged liver has difficulty breaking down proteins, raw proteins such as those found in sushi (eaten without the rice) and sashimi are healthy for the liver. The raw fish is loaded with enzymes and is less stressful because it is raw rather than cooked. Cooked fish is the next best thing, then chicken and lamb. Eggs are also good unless the gallbladder is sluggish.

Red meats tend to be a bit more stressful to digest than fish, but in small quantities they are fine. A large cooked piece of meat is very stressful on the liver. As far as red meat is concerned, it's much easier for the liver to digest a rare steak than a fully cooked one. However, don't ask for a "rare" burger at the McDonald's drive-up window. I'm talking about a high-quality steak. A small amount of red meat would be okay a few times per week; but when you add the bun to the hamburger, it creates more stress on the liver.

In college, I don't think I ate even one vegetable. I told myself, "I'll eat healthy when I graduate." Boy, was that smart! Shortly after graduating I started getting liver symptoms and it took a long time for me to recover. To this day I still don't enjoy vegetables, but they are mainstays of my diet because now I know better.

I had one patient from the Philippines who lost 42 pounds of water weight from his stomach within six weeks of doing my program. Depending on the size of the belly, it could take two to six months to completely flatten the stomach; fat comes off gradually, while fluid weight can come off rapidly. But the potbelly comes off to the degree that you create a healthy liver.

You can't take a person who has a lifetime of poor eating and expect two weeks of healthy eating to fix the liver. Unless you've been eating organic foods, the chances are good that you have been ingesting foods exposed to pesticides, insecticides, antibiotics, herbicides, fungicides and estrogen.

If a person has liver damage, cholesterol accumulation will usually occur, primarily because the liver is the main organ that breaks it down.[8] Lots of my patients with high cholesterol and even high blood pressure see excellent results from our eating plan. In fact, this plan is beneficial for anyone who has high cholesterol.

Here's one success story that was sent to the person's medical doctor:

> "It is this program that enabled me to lower my cholesterol from 226 to 197. My triglycerides also dropped from 104 to 64 during the same testing period. Similarly, my wife's cholesterol dropped from 248 to 187. Basically our carbs come from fresh dark-green vegetables. We are eating at least 4 ounces of animal protein with every meal, including eggs and hormone-free meats (chicken, fish, pork and beef). We eat virtually no grains, bread or pasta and have very little processed sugar intake. Additionally, I have lost 20 pounds since I started with the regimen."
>
> —RR, Centerville, VA

Cholesterol and Eggs

Since we are on the topic of cholesterol, you should know about the antidote (remedy) to cholesterol—lecithin. Rather than only avoiding cholesterol foods, it would be better to make sure you include foods high in lecithin. And you might be surprised that a very excellent source of lecithin is the egg yolk—the exact thing people who have high cholesterol are told to avoid. Even the derivation of *lecithin*, the Greek word *lekithos*, means "yolk of an egg." Eating eggs with yolks is beneficial for the liver, not only because of the high lecithin, but because they are a complete balanced food and easy to digest. However, if you have a sluggish gallbladder, fish would be a better source of protein. Gallbladder symptoms give you right-shoulder pain, fullness in the right lower-abdomen area and burping and belching after you eat. Personally, I eat a 4-ounce piece of fish for breakfast—it might sound strange, but my body runs better on that than other proteins. Twice a week I will have eggs.

Atherosclerosis

While on the subject of cholesterol, let me tell you my theory on what causes atherosclerosis (so-called clogged arteries). People have this idea that when they eat excessive fatty foods the cholesterol floats around in their arteries and starts to plug them up. This is not what happens. The plaque occurs not on the inside of the artery but within the inner lining of the artery. So it must be more an internal problem than cholesterol floating and plugging. Some other credible authors believe that what initiates this is a breakdown within the artery wall.[9]

The arteries are made of collagen, which is a protein. Therefore, hormones that destroy proteins must be involved in the process (excess cortisol and deficiency of growth hormone). This could be the reason people with adrenal problems bruise easily. Repair and maintenance of these arteries also require vitamin C. That is why people with vitamin C deficiencies get weaknesses within the blood vessels, as in bleeding gums, spider veins and varicose veins. Vitamin C helps in the formation of the collagen, or cement, that holds everything together. Vitamin E is the other vitamin that assists in the repair of tissues—it is the healing vitamin. I personally believe that in a vitamin C and E deficient state the person is very susceptible to atherosclerosis. Mushrooms provide an excellent source of vitamin C. Raw wheat germ is an excellent source of vitamin E; however, you don't need much—one teaspoon three times per week. Leafy green vegetables are the foods that contain both these vitamins.

Liver Spots

This leads to another topic—liver or aging spots, usually on the backs of the hands. There are many theories about this. My theory is that a vitamin E deficiency has something to do with creating this brown pigment. It could also come from the destruction of certain liver cells that make the pigment. Another cause could be a deficiency in a hormone from the pituitary gland in the brain that triggers the color of the skin.

What's interesting about this is that a good portion of the body's vitamin E is stored in the pituitary gland. That is because it is needed for making hormones, especially all the sex hormones in the ovaries—estrogen, testosterone, etc. During menopause when the ovaries shut down, a woman's vitamin E levels dramatically decrease due to the altered pituitary-ovary connection; and when the liver loses its vitamin E supply, a brown pigment gets released. I would recommend all women over the age of 50 consume a half-teaspoon of raw wheat germ every day to keep their vitamin E at a normal level. Wheat-germ oil also works.

Growth Hormone

Growth hormone (GH) is directly associated with the liver and works through the liver. It is fat-burning and anti-aging; it also controls the rebuilding of joints. A bad liver can prevent growth hormone from being produced. This shows up in excess fat, less lean body mass and squeaky joints (to put it technically).

I'm sure you have heard the hype on how GH is the fountain of youth. Growth hormone makes children's bones grow, regulates the size of your organs, decreases fat (fat-burning), increases lean body mass, and controls sleep cycles the first half of the night. It rebuilds body tissue: joints, bone and muscle. Other hormones break down these proteins—for instance, the adrenal stress hormone cortisol.

Cortisol, if in excess, will eat up your thigh muscles, making it difficult to climb stairs or get up from a chair. In many cases, it's not growth hormone that is the problem but the cortisol that inhibits it. Years of stress, lack of sleep, bad foods, low-calorie diets, hard-core exercise, pain, inflammation and overactive adrenal glands can block growth hormone.

Many people take growth hormone without ever first finding out why they might be deficient—a poor liver. Growth hormone is made to protect, spare or save muscle, bone and joint proteins from being destroyed while at the same time keeping the fuel adequate between meals. The pancreas hormone insulin regulates fuel when you eat. Growth hormone regulates fuel between meals.

Since growth hormone is stimulated when you are not eating, we recommend consuming only two to three meals per day.

Another activity that helps GH is exercise—not just any old exercise but intense exercise. There seems to be a direct relationship between growth hormone and the intensity of exercise, especially weight training and short, quick, intense types of sports. The problem is that cortisol is stimulated by stress and cortisol inhibits growth hormone. The trick is to trigger growth hormone without triggering cortisol. This means you need to do high-intensity, short-duration exercise with lots of rest in between. You'll learn more about this in chapter 17. Getting enough sleep also triggers growth hormone, and for this reason fat burning occurs during sleep.

We've discussed what increases GH. Now let me mention what you need to avoid in order to prevent a decrease in GH. Sugar blocks GH. It's not sugar directly but the hormone that is triggered by sugar—insulin. Insulin is the fat-making hormone. Insulin changes carbohydrates (sugar) into fat and cholesterol. When insulin rises, growth hormone is blocked. This is why a belly full of carbohydrates before bed will inhibit GH from working through the night.[10] Even a small glass of juice or wine will prevent growth hormone through the night. I'm sorry, but that's the way it is.

Don't eat carbs at least 90 minutes before bed, especially the sweet ones. This includes hidden carbs such as beer, flavored yogurt and breads. You'd be shocked to find out what food manufacturers put sugar in these days—start reading labels and you'll see. You would burn more fat if you didn't eat anything before bed. I'm not saying never, but the more you stick to this, the more quickly fat will be burned. If you're going to drink, drink your alcohol in the morning (just kidding). Consuming carbs like juice, sugary sports drinks or so-called protein bars one hour before you work out can block growth hormone as well. I wouldn't even recommend eating fruit before working out.

Some of us just don't have time to sleep. I've had patients who get only three to four hours routinely. Getting less than seven hours per night can inhibit fat-burning hormones. If you are having sleep problems, there are several things you can do. Long walks during the daylight, reading a book before bed instead of watching TV, taking a calcium supplement (calcium with magnesium citrate), doing physical work around the yard, especially if you sit behind a computer screen, and consuming four celery sticks before bed are all good remedies.

Some research has found initial benefits from taking growth hormone: subjects on GH lost an average of 14.4 percent body fat and gained 8.8 percent lean body mass without diet or exercise.[11] The problem was that after several months of being on growth hormone, major side effects began: carpal tunnel syndrome, fluid retention, high blood pressure, joint pain, high blood sugar, diabetes, cancer, and inflammation in the pancreas.[12] This is because when you bypass your body's own production of GH, your body's production starts to decrease. Go ahead and take it if you have eight months to live. Other than that, I wouldn't recommend it.

A problem with the liver can often prevent it from making enough bile. Bile is the fluid that helps you break down fats AND absorb fat-soluble vitamins (A, D, E and K). Adding Gallbladder Formula (one after each meal) can help replace what's missing, especially if you are missing the gallbladder itself. This product supplies purified bile salts and many additional factors to support a healthy gallbladder (see Resources section).

I want to emphasize that when one has no gallbladder, bile merely trickles down a tube (bile duct) from the liver directly into the small intestine; whereas if you have a gallbladder, you secrete a much larger amount of bile when you eat. The gallbladder, when full, is the size of a small potato. Also, it concentrates bile by five times. So with a healthy gallbladder, not only are you getting more release of bile, but a much stronger concentration of bile is being released.

Key Indicators

Key Liver type indicators are potbelly, brown spots on the backs of hands, yellowness in the whites of eyes, and poor joints. (See diagram on the next page.)

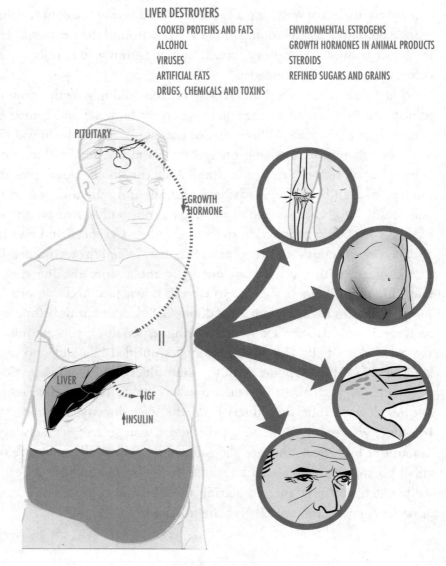

LIVER DESTROYERS

COOKED PROTEINS AND FATS
ALCOHOL
VIRUSES
ARTIFICIAL FATS
DRUGS, CHEMICALS AND TOXINS

ENVIRONMENTAL ESTROGENS
GROWTH HORMONES IN ANIMAL PRODUCTS
STEROIDS
REFINED SUGARS AND GRAINS

PITUITARY

GROWTH HORMONE

LIVER

↓IGF

↑INSULIN

COMMON LIVER ISSUES

IGF: Insulin-like growth factor. For more information on this hormone, see chapter 3, page 33, under "Fat-Burning Hormones," and chapter 9, page 127, under "Trigger #3."

Below is a list of symptoms the Liver type can experience from a poorly working liver.

Liver Type Symptoms

- Potbelly (very little external fat, mostly fluid)
- Brown spots on backs of hands and throughout body
- Poor joints
- Yellowness in whites of eyes (severe cases)
- Bloodshot eyes in the morning
- Eyelids itchy and swollen
- Hives and itchiness
- Skin problems
- Little red dots on skin
- Bloating after eating
- Burping or belching after eating
- Acid reflux
- Constipation
- Hemorrhoids
- Decreased tolerance for fatty foods and refined grains
- Cravings for fried foods and sour foods
- Chemical sensitivities
- Stiffness in lower back and upper back between the shoulder blades
- Pain or tightness in right-shoulder area
- Liver roll of fat (just below the rib cage), seen mostly in women
- Dull pressure and sensation of fullness just under right rib cage
- Gallbladder problems
- Headaches
- Arthritis
- High cholesterol
- High blood pressure
- Varicose veins
- Spider veins
- Bad breath
- Tongue coated with white film

- Deep split down center of tongue
- Early-morning insomnia (wake up one to two hours before alarm)
- Irritability and moodiness, especially in the morning
- Foggy brain in the morning
- Finger joints stiff, sore and swollen in the morning
- Fingers clubbed, with whitened nail beds
- Urine darker in morning, getting clearer during day
- Light-colored bowel movements
- Swelling in ankles
- Overheating of body, especially hot feet at night (not hot flashes)

9

The 10 Fat-Burning Triggers and Blockers

There are two basic types of problems with weight that need to be addressed: (1) fat and (2) water weight.

The first, actual fat, is a problem of a failing endocrine system (glands and hormones).

The second, fluid retention, is a problem of sodium and potassium imbalance, which could also be failing endocrine glands—adrenals. Fixing both of these problems requires avoiding what has created them in the first place. Then actions need to be taken to restore glandular health. It's not just a matter of triggering your fat-burning hormones but, more importantly, avoiding those things that prevent fat burning and proper mineral balance. If you trigger fat-burning hormones without keeping the fat-making hormones to a minimum, you won't lose any weight, since all fat burners are nullified in the presence of fat-making hormones.

There are many ways you can attempt to lose weight. The high-protein, low-carbohydrate diets will help lower insulin but fail to balance sodium and potassium ratios. Potassium is needed to support fat-burning hormones. Low-calorie diets, on the other hand, will help temporary weight loss but will activate adrenal stress hormones, causing a rebound with a slower metabolism and more weight down the road. Low-fat diets can starve the body of raw materials for building fat-burning hormones, as these are made out of fat. High-fat diets can aggravate the liver, which is needed for all the six fat-burning hormones to work. High vegetable and fruit diets help with proper sodium and potassium ratios but fail to give enough protein to stimulate fat burning. The moderation diet of vegetables, so-called healthy whole grains and proteins is also not workable as far as hormones are concerned because "eating everything in moderation" (whole-grain foods, juice, wine or sugar) can block fat burning very easily.

In this program we will be smarter, by taking as many actions as possible to support hormone health while avoiding things that destroy hormone function.

Below are the ten very important factors in achieving this goal.

Trigger #1

The Absence of Sugar

Of all the things that have an impact on your metabolism, the most important one is sugar. Sugar triggers the powerful fat-making, fat-storing hormone insulin. In fact, in the presence of insulin not only will fat be blocked from being used as fuel BUT sugar will be converted to fat.

Sugar is a carbohydrate. And the most powerful trigger to fat burning is "the absence of sugar."

If given the choice of what it likes as a fuel source, the body will ALWAYS choose sugar as a preferred fuel over fat.[1] *This means that in order to burn fat, you can't have any sugar in the diet.*

Hidden sugars include vanilla yogurt or flavored yogurt, gum, alcohol, wine, beer, juice (especially orange juice), sports drinks, sodas, salad dressing with sugar, desserts, and even ketchup with high-fructose corn syrup. Many people have no idea of the number of hidden sugars in their diets.

Some people will try to convince you that chocolate and wine have powerful health benefits as antioxidants. Yet the amount of damage to your glands far outweighs any benefits from these antioxidants.

Other hidden sugars include **refined grains**, such as cereal, pasta, breads, crackers, pretzels, muffins, cakes, cookies, pancakes, waffles, donuts, rice cakes and puffed-rice cereals.

People have a big confusion about grains, which is contributed to greatly by promotion from the food industry: *Consume healthy whole-wheat grains instead of refined grains.* It doesn't matter if it's whole-wheat or white bread; these starches turn into sugar fairly rapidly. Many people are also allergic to them, which leads to water retention and digestive troubles. I have found that cutting out grains is a very important factor in getting someone into fat burning. The only acceptable grain product in small amounts would be bran (the outer shell of the grain), which is high in fiber. Vegetable fiber is better quality because it has more nutrition, but fiber in general does slow the insulin hormone response.

Vegetable starches are also converted to fat. These would include potatoes, yams, corn, potato chips, french fries, hash browns, corn chips, etc.

And then there are the **fruits: melons and berries** have a higher sugar content than vegetable carbohydrates and will trigger insulin; although the fiber they contain acts as a buffer, slightly slowing this response. **Bananas, dates, figs, raisins, canned fruit, dried fruits and mangoes** also have a high sugar content but with lower fiber, and these have a much greater effect on insulin. In the previous edition of this book I recommended apples and other fruits. However, fruit can stop weight loss, particularly if your metabolism is slow. Do not consume any fruits if you are trying to lose weight, especially apples; an apple contains 19 grams of sugar and will surely stop weight loss. (Some fruits might not cause weight gain but they can certainly prevent weight loss from occurring.) Once you hit your goal, though, you can add them back into your diet. The only exception to this rule is including a small amount (one cup) of berries in your kale shake. Most people can get away with eating one cup of berries per day.

When you eliminate **sugary foods** like ice cream, candy, chocolate, added sugar to coffee and tea, and canned fruit with syrup, your body can tap into fat burning because the trigger for fat release is *the absence of sugar*.[2]

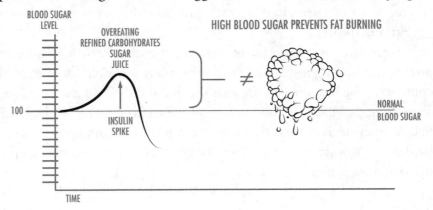

BLOOD SUGAR LEVEL

OVEREATING
REFINED CARBOHYDRATES
SUGAR
JUICE

HIGH BLOOD SUGAR PREVENTS FAT BURNING

≠

100

INSULIN SPIKE

NORMAL BLOOD SUGAR

TIME

All aspects of fat burning are enhanced by the absence of sugar.[3] Cut out sugar as well as those foods that turn quickly into sugar and you'll automatically trigger fat-burning hormones. The best sugar substitute is the herb stevia (I recommend clear stevia). The next best sweeteners are erythritol, xylitol or other sugar alcohol sweeteners. However, start out light, as they may have a laxative effect; although for most people this is not an issue. Make sure they are non-GMO. Do not consume honey, agave or fructose. When sugar is not consumed, another hormone is triggered called glucagon. Glucagon does the opposite of insulin.[4] If insulin makes you fat, glucagon makes you thin. Glucagon is also triggered by protein (an adequate amount) and exercise.

The body has only a very small capacity to store sugar; anything over that will be automatically converted and stored as fat and cholesterol. To store sugar, potassium is needed. Without potassium, sugar storage is greatly limited and fat storing is enhanced. Sugar cane normally has lots of potassium, but when it's refined, potassium is lost. Therefore, if a person consumes refined white sugar, which is void of potassium, the body will store less sugar and make more fat and cholesterol.

Let me further clarify this by stating it another way: When the diet is deficient in potassium, the body is forced to store more fat than sugar; whereas when there is adequate dietary potassium, the body will store the sugar and convert less of it to fat.

Refined sugar also triggers sodium and water retention by decreasing potassium (opposing mineral).

Potassium is a body relaxer and calms the pulse rate. Since eating refined sugar depletes potassium, this increases the pulse rate, which you might have experienced as a pulsating pounding in the ears when you were trying to sleep.

If there is even a little bit of sugar in the diet, or if insulin is kept just slightly too high, fat fuel cannot be made available for energy. You could have the best diet throughout the day and then eat a small piece of something sweet at night and nullify all the good eating. With bad eating habits a person is constantly playing catch-up by working out twice as hard tomorrow or saying, "I'll eat better the next day to make up the damage from today."

Sugar will additionally block the fat-burning effects of exercise. For example, drinking a small amount of juice prior to exercising blocks the fat-burning hormones (especially growth hormone).[5]

In order for the diet to be successful, sugar needs to be completely eliminated. Once your body is healthy and you reach your ideal weight, then it will be able to tolerate occasional sugars, but not until you achieve your goal. Even drinking wine at night can set your liver back a few days.

Many people might not realize that the fat on their bodies actually comes from the sugar they eat, not from the fat they eat.

The same is true of cholesterol. Many people have high cholesterol not because they are consuming a lot of bacon or heavy fats but because they are eating large quantities of refined grains, sugars and starches.

This is a result of the influence of hormones over foods.

As you age, the conversion of sugar into fat increases, making it very difficult to get away with any sugars. This has to do with the combination of a slower metabolism and aging organs, as well as hormone shifts. If you're younger, you can get away with eating poorly . . . well, at least temporarily; but over the age of 40, watch out. You can *look* at a sugar cube and bam! Ten pounds! If you're young and reading this, learn from the mistakes of others.

Excess sugar mixed with excess protein greatly increases insulin (fat-making hormone).[6] Sugary dessert after a large steak will increase insulin in a big way. Some other examples of this are BBQ Buffalo wings that contain sugar, breaded meats, meatloaf, ham, some deli meats that contain dextrose, or meat and potatoes. Protein without sugar only triggers insulin slightly; however, protein in general activates two other fat burners—glucagon and growth hormone.[7]

Insulin is the principal hormone triggered by refined carbohydrates and sugar. It is also a key hormone that stores fat. In the presence of any insulin, ALL other fat-burning hormones are nullified and blocked. So, not only is fat burning suppressed but fat is produced.

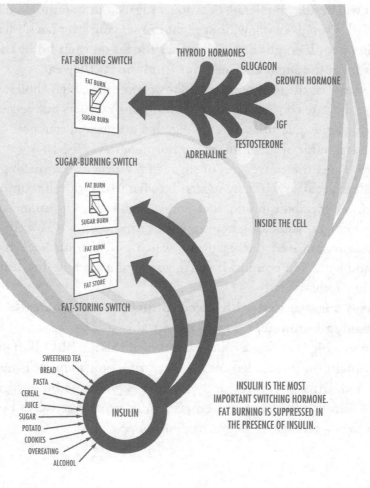

Trigger #2

Vegetables

Vegetable: *n.* of the plant family compared to the animal family. [Latin *vegetare*, "to enliven" < *vegetus*, "lively" < *vegere*, "to quicken," "wake." Late Latin *vegetabilis*, "animating"]

There are several important reasons why I included vegetables (non-starchy) in these triggers.

If the cause of your weight problem is a sick or failing endocrine system, then we need some nutrient-dense live food to heal it. The vegetable family has several qualities that aid in healing. Eaten raw, vegetables are one of the most concentrated sources of vitamins, minerals and plant chemicals. They are high in fiber, which buffers the fat maker insulin. They are also low in sugar, even though they are called a carbohydrate.

Heat destroys nutrients. If the goal is to heal your body, then the more raw vegetables you eat, the faster this process will occur. Cooked vegetables will take away from the healing process. If you steam your vegetables, make sure they are lightly steamed, and also eat raw vegetables during the day. Ideally, you would consume 80 percent raw vegetables.

Vegetables have excellent ratios of high potassium and very low sodium. On the following page is a short list of high-potassium foods in milligrams. If you look at this chart, you can see that vegetables in general have very little sodium and high amounts of potassium. However, there are some vegetables that have high levels of sodium as well as high levels of potassium, such as beets and celery. These vegetables are beneficial for people with calcium deposits in their bodies, like gallstones and kidney stones, as sodium helps to balance the excess calcium.

The majority of overweight people are severely dehydrated in their cells and waterlogged outside their cells *despite* drinking lots of water. It sometimes takes up to six months of eating lots of vegetables to replace the potassium within the cells. You have to get it from food; taking a potassium supplement can't correct this problem. Processed, refined, boxed and canned foods do just the reverse: they create fluid retention because of the high sodium and low potassium.

Food	Amount	Potassium (mg)	Sodium (mg)
Apple	1 medium	158.70	0.00
Asparagus	1 cup	288.00	19.80
Avocado	1 cup	874.54	14.60
Banana	1 medium	467.28	1.18
Beef	4 oz	475.15	71.44
Beet	1 cup	518.50	484.50
Blackstrap Molasses	2 tsp	340.57	7.52
Broccoli	1 cup	505.44	42.12
Brussels Sprouts	1 cup	494.52	32.76
Cabbage	1 cup	145.50	12.00
Cantaloupe	1 cup	494.40	14.40
Carrot	1 cup	394.06	42.70
Cauliflower	1 cup	176.08	18.60
Celery	1 cup	344.40	103.40
Cranberries	½ cup	33.73	0.47
Grapefruit	½	158.67	0.00
Honey	1 oz	22.04	1.70
Kale	1 cup	296.40	29.90
Kidney Beans	1 cup	713.31	3.54
Lemon/Lime	¼ cup	75.64	0.61
Milk	1 cup	376.74	121.76
Mushrooms (crimini)	1 cup	635.04	8.51
Potato (with skin)	1 cup	509.96	9.76
Romaine Lettuce	1 cup	324.80	8.96
Rye	1 cup	148.72	3.38
Salmon	4 oz	572.67	68.04
Tomato	1 cup	399.60	16.20
Walnuts	¼ cup	110.25	0.50
Watermelon	1 cup	176.32	3.04

The nutrient profiles provided in the above chart are derived from
Food Processor for Windows, Version 7.60, by ESHA Research in Salem, Oregon, USA.

At my clinic we have a device that measures body fat and fluid levels, and the most startling breakthrough on this subject has been the discovery that many male patients coming into our office weighing between 250 and 350 pounds have normal or only slightly above normal body fat. However, they are full of fluid; and when someone has more fluid than fat, their sodium to potassium ratios are usually off. This is why we need lots of veggies each day (7 to 10 cups), as these foods are high in potassium, which will slowly bring the body fluid levels into a normal range. This works when you address the problem with whole foods. It doesn't work when you try to handle it with supplements. Any water weight problems always need high-potassium foods.

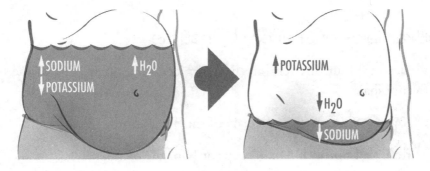

INCREASING POTASSIUM WILL DECREASE SODIUM AND WATER

Potassium helps lower insulin. Without enough potassium, your insulin could increase and keep you out of fat burning. Potassium is also needed to adequately hold protein in your body (especially in the muscles). The electrical charge and energy of your cells are dependent upon incoming potassium. The best source of potassium, better than bananas, is vegetables.

Each day our bodies require 4,000 to 4,700 milligrams of potassium. That's a lot, and I encourage you to consume 7 to 10 cups of salad or vegetables per day to get close to this amount. You can also obtain potassium from your meats; so if we total up what I am recommending, you should hit your requirement of potassium. Adding this change to your diet will be one of the most significant health-creating actions of your life. It might seem impossible, but after you try it, you'll feel so good!

Just have two large salads a day—or, like me, ONE HUGE salad at lunch. If this is too difficult, then drink your salad as a shake by combining kale and a small quantity of berries (1 cup). However, if your metabolism is slow, I would leave out the berries and instead add 10 drops of liquid berry-flavored stevia. (See the kale shake recipe below.)

> The only problem is that a small number of people bloat when they consume the kale shake. If this happens to you, switch to spinach or consume salads. You're not going to lose weight if you're bloating. Another trick I use for this is blending the kale shake and storing it in the refrigerator overnight, then drinking it the next morning. Allowing it to sit overnight in the refrigerator lets the fibers break down a bit, which is easier on the digestive system.

Examples of Shakes I Consume

Here are four different greens and green mixes that I use as the base for my shakes:

Kale or Spinach (3 cups or ½ of the blender full)

Kale and Spinach Mix (3 cups or ½ of the blender full)

Kale and Parsley Mix (3 cups or ½ of the blender full)

Kale, Parsley and Beet Tops (3 cups or ½ of the blender full)
    MY FAVORITE!

To each of the greens I add the following:
• 1 cup berries
• 2 Tbsp lemon juice
Fill with water (just above ingredients in blender).
Blend for 4 minutes.

I store my kale, spinach and parsley in bags in the freezer so they last longer. Also, frozen vegetables blend better.

Cruciferous Vegetables

Cruciferous vegetables have some very interesting properties; they are anti-estrogen, anti-cancer, anti–toxic chemical, and greatly help the liver in its ability to detoxify. Because estrogen is fat making and blocks the fat-burning growth hormone, eating many of these vegetables can help weight loss.

- Cabbage
- Brussels sprouts
- Broccoli
- Cauliflower
- Kale
- Radishes
- Turnips and turnip greens
- Bok choy
- Watercress
- Collards
- Mustard greens
- Rutabaga

Many people are told that consuming cruciferous vegetables will deplete their iodine reserves, thus worsening their thyroid glands. If you consume a good amount of cruciferous vegetables in your diet, the best solution is to merely add some iodine from sea kelp. Sea kelp, if grown in a healthy part of the world, can provide not just iodine but all the trace minerals—and in plant form for easier absorption. Sea kelp also contains selenium, which is essential for the conversion of thyroid hormones—to make sure that T4 gets activated into T3. (See Resources section for more information on sea kelp.)

The benefits of cruciferous vegetables far outweigh any negatives. Cruciferous vegetables help balance an excess-estrogen situation, which is one of the causes of hypothyroidism—an underactive thyroid gland. The ONLY reason I would avoid cruciferous vegetables is if you experience bloating. In this case, steam them or cook them until no more bloating occurs. Personally, I cannot consume broccoli, as it will cause severe cramps; however, I can eat kale with no problem.

Trigger #3

Protein

Protein is a powerful trigger for fat-burning hormones if it's not in excess. Protein stimulates two hormones—glucagon and growth hormone. Now, there are two factors that should be discussed.

The first one involves the amount of protein. If you eat too much protein, insulin (fat-making hormone) can be triggered. Excess protein can create almost the same insulin response as refined carbohydrates. And another point that is new for many people is the fact that the leaner the protein— the less fat it has—the greater the insulin response. More on this later.

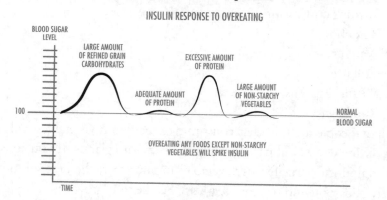

INSULIN RESPONSE TO OVEREATING

BLOOD SUGAR LEVEL

LARGE AMOUNT OF REFINED GRAIN CARBOHYDRATES

EXCESSIVE AMOUNT OF PROTEIN

ADEQUATE AMOUNT OF PROTEIN

LARGE AMOUNT OF NON-STARCHY VEGETABLES

100

NORMAL BLOOD SUGAR

OVEREATING ANY FOODS EXCEPT NON-STARCHY VEGETABLES WILL SPIKE INSULIN

TIME

Your body can only absorb a maximum of 35 grams of protein at one sitting; this is about 5 to 6 ounces of steak. Anything extra has a tendency to be converted to sugar-spiking insulin, especially if it's lean protein or low-fat protein or protein powder (whey). *But please note that 35 grams is the limit only if you have a healthy liver. Most people with resistant weight have unhealthy livers and can't digest even close to that in one sitting.* So, with liver problems, eat less protein. Also, if the thyroid is slow, the liver will not be able to process large amounts of protein.

I no longer recommend eating more frequent protein meals, four to five times per day. Why? Because insulin gets released anytime you eat. These extra spikes of insulin throughout the day will guarantee you never lose weight. Avoid snacking between meals and add more healthy fats during the other meals.

IGF stands for insulin-like growth factor, which is a hormone the liver produces to regulate blood sugars between meals by releasing stored fuel (such as fat). It works in a similar way to growth hormone and is even triggered by GH.

If the liver is damaged and this hormone can't work, the pancreas is forced to pump out more insulin, which could lead to diabetes. So insulin and IGF work in tandem, insulin regulating the blood sugars during meals and IGF regulating blood sugars between meals.

Each body type responds differently to dietary protein. The liver is the hub of digestion, and if the liver is dysfunctional, it is very easy to overdo it by eating excessive protein, especially cooked protein. If you have a Liver body type, eat less protein (3 ounces per meal) so as not to stress the liver. Adjust your proteins to smaller amounts and also consume proteins that are not cooked as much—as in rare steak, or eggs with the yolk runny, or even raw fish (tartare).

If you have an Adrenal body type, then you need more protein. Why? Because the adrenal glands tend to destroy proteins, by breaking down muscles, faster than other body types. You'll need to replace the destroyed protein with dietary proteins (3 to 6 ounces).

The Thyroid body type has such a slow metabolism that protein is more difficult to digest. Thyroid cases do well with small amounts of protein (3 ounces per meal).

The Ovary body type, with its high estrogen, needs a moderate amount of protein (3 to 6 ounces).

The second important factor with protein is consuming it in its whole form. Just as there are refined carbohydrates, there are also refined proteins. These include protein powders and protein bars. Protein powder is always lean and low-fat and interestingly will spike insulin more than whole-food protein, which comes with fat. If I do make a shake with low-fat protein powder, I add some fat to it. Proteins in their whole state are best: whole eggs, whole-milk cheese, non-lean meat, fish, and chicken with the skin on.

Consuming overly cooked protein can also be hard on the glands. This would include overdone beef, sausage, hot dogs, too many roasted nuts, milk (pasteurized) and excessive peanut butter. If you eat peanut butter, you may need some digestive help (Gallbladder Formula). I find that almond butter is much healthier. And if you eat cooked protein, balance it out with lots of vegetables too. Yogurt, kefir and cheese are fermented and/or cultured and are considered partially raw; they have live enzymes. Yet even plain yogurt contains quite a bit of sugar; so hold off on this right now. Plain kefir is okay to eat occasionally. Cheese, on the other hand, is lower in sugar and not a problem on this program. Of course, you wouldn't eat raw chicken meat. Hard-boiled eggs are okay to eat anytime.

Amino acids are the building blocks of protein. The amino acids arginine, glycine, tryptophan and valine are powerful stimulators of fat-burning hormones.[8] Instead of taking these in supplement form, why not get them from foods? You will notice that the foods recommended in this program contain highly concentrated fat-burning amino acids. These amino acids are present in Brie cheese, kefir, avocado, coconut, pecans, walnuts, almonds, Brazil nuts, hazelnuts, pine nuts, pumpkin seeds, sesame seeds, sunflower seeds, beef, poultry (chicken and turkey), wild game (pheasant, quail), seafood (halibut, lobster, salmon, shrimp, snails, tuna in water), eggs, chickpeas, winter squash and mushrooms.

Protein can increase the fat on your body, but only if consumed in large quantities (9 to 12+ ounces). The recommended protein consumption by the government is way too high. However, some of the protein you eat is not used for fuel but is used to replace body proteins—muscles, bone, cells, and so on.[9]

One last point regarding animal proteins has to do with their quality. Consume organic (without hormones), grass-fed meat and wild-caught fish rather than commercial grain-fed meat and farm-raised fish. The cancer-protective properties of healthy omega fatty acid ratios are much better, and for the body to heal, omega fats are necessary in their correct ratios.

There is an interesting point on collagen, a protein that is found in skin, joints, vertebral discs, ligaments, tendons, and so on: If you have loose skin, weak joints and back, brittle nails, splitting hair, and even hair loss, you would think you merely needed to increase your dietary protein to resolve these issues. Yet most of the time this won't work. That's because the real problem is rarely a lack of protein. There can be several other causes: (1) Loss of trace minerals (minerals required in small amounts); minerals and trace minerals are intimately involved with the formation of protein through biochemical enzymes. (2) Higher levels of the stress hormone cortisol, which is very destructive against proteins. (3) Lack of stomach acids; it takes a very acidic stomach to break down protein, and if your stomach is not acidic enough, you'll experience a loss of collagen, gas, indigestion, heartburn, and even GERD (gastroesophageal reflux disorder, or acid reflux).* (4) Being a diabetic or prediabetic, which can block body proteins needed for muscle growth, due to the insulin required for protein formation.

Trigger #4

Fats

Fats typically do not influence fat-making hormones; however, they do have the ability to stress the liver and gallbladder, which indirectly affects hormone flows through the liver.

This is why too many fatty nuts cause your right shoulder, shoulder blade and neck to hurt. The three-pound liver under the right side of your chest can swell and irritate the right shoulder.

The whole myth that fat is the big culprit that is making everyone fat doesn't pan out when you're talking about hormones. Fat has little effect on fat-storing hormones. Many people put too much importance on restricting fats in the diet. Yes, it is true that with Liver types low fats are best; however, this is not because fat turns into fat, but because fat stresses the liver. Fat is also necessary to allow you to go longer without eating. If you are a prediabetic or have blood sugar issues, which so many people do, it's necessary to not snack between meals, and this is another reason to add more satiating fat.

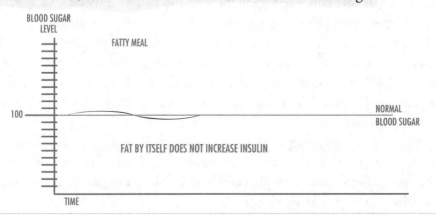

---

* See Resources section for nutrient recommendations for trace minerals and Digest Formula.

There are also studies showing that a low-fat diet inhibits the fat-burning hormone testosterone. This is why you need to include nuts, seeds, avocados, flax oil and olive oil in your diet, as well as the other fats listed in this section.

What most people don't understand is that carbohydrates (breads, sugars, wine, juice, etc.) are changed into fat and cholesterol much more readily than fat and cholesterol foods are turned into adipose tissue and increased blood cholesterol. In other words, low-fat cookies will make fat and cholesterol faster than cholesterol-laden eggs will. And eggs are rich in the antidote to cholesterol—lecithin. The other point is that eggs will increase ONLY your good cholesterol, not the bad.

Did you realize that your body makes 3,000 milligrams of cholesterol in your liver and cells every day? Yes, it does. That is equivalent to the amount of cholesterol which is present in 333 strips of bacon or one pound of butter or 14 eggs. Our bodies use a ton of cholesterol for hormones and body tissue.

An important point to know about cholesterol is that when dietary intake of cholesterol foods is high, the body will make less, and when dietary cholesterol intake is low, the body will make more.[10] This explains why many people still have high cholesterol despite consuming less of it.

It is also often not understood that cholesterol is only present in animal products and is not found in nuts, avocados, seeds or olives.

Another interesting factor concerning fat and cholesterol is that a good portion of your body is made of fat—brain, nerves, hormones and glands. Your body is constantly replacing these tissues with dietary fats. So, despite fats having more calories per gram compared with carbohydrates, some of these fats are used to replace body parts. This is especially true under stress, as the adrenals need to build more stress hormones. Carbohydrates are not used to replace body parts but are used only for fuel and vitamin and mineral supply. This is why excess carbohydrates are readily converted to fat as storage.

Hormonally speaking, eating carbohydrates is much more devastating for weight gain than the consumption of fat; and some studies even show that you will lose more weight on a high-fat, low-carbohydrate diet than on a low-fat, high-carbohydrate diet.[11]

Satisfying Effect

Cravings come from letting your blood sugars drop too low. When you eat fats, hormones are triggered to make you feel satisfied and eliminate the cravings. Carbohydrates, on the other hand, will not trigger these hormones but will do the opposite and inhibit the satisfying effect, causing more hunger. This is why eating sugar and refined carbohydrates will create a desire to consume more an hour later. Many people are eating the wrong foods, which keeps them craving and hungry all the time. Eggs—especially with the yolks—raw nuts, avocados and cheese are excellent foods to stimulate certain hormones and to decrease hunger and cravings.[12]

Two Types of Fuel

There are two types of fuel: fat and sugar.

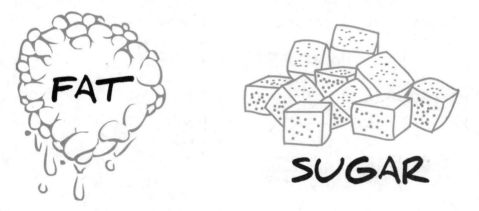

The body, if healthy, can switch from one to the other. Most people are switched to only sugar burning. Fat fuel is the most satisfying. Burning only sugar will eventually cause a problem with the hormone that regulates sugar: insulin. Your cells will start to block and resist incoming insulin. If the cells can't get sugar fuel, the cells are never satisfied because they can't eat despite how much food is being eaten. They develop a condition called *insulin resistance.*

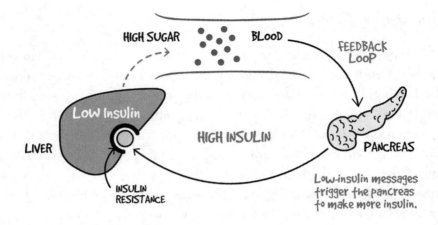

Low-insulin messages trigger the pancreas to make more insulin.

INSULIN RESISTANCE is a prediabetic condition whereby the cells (liver, muscles, brain, etc.) are resisting insulin. This triggers blood sugars to rise and also prevents fuel from entering the cells because insulin remains low in the blood. The feedback from the blood causes the pancreas to make more.

Insulin not only has the function of lowering sugar in the blood, but it also acts as a key to open the cells to fuel (glucose).

HOW DOES INSULIN WORK?

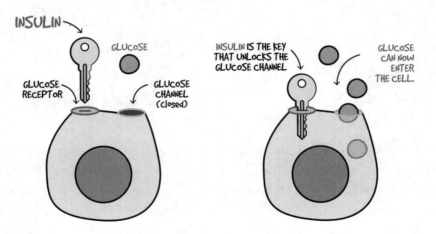

Hungry Cells That Can't Eat

If your cells are not absorbing fuel or nutrition, they will not be satisfied. This triggers the brain to crave sweets and seek out sweets. The bad part of this is that a person with insulin resistance has five to seven times more insulin than a normal person. This means there is plenty of insulin but it's dysfunctional insulin—it can't work.

However, when we switch the body over to fat burning by keeping insulin low, we can avoid the high and low blood sugar swings, which keep us craving, tired and cranky, with brain fog. In summary, if insulin is low, we burn fat; when insulin is high, we burn sugar.

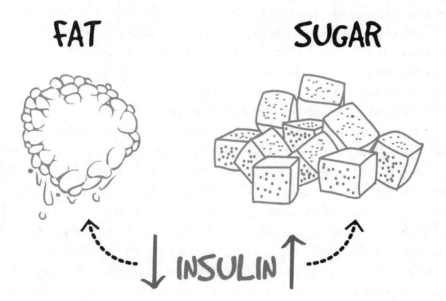

Essential Fats

Essential fats are fats that are vital to the body yet cannot be made by the body. These essential fatty acids, as they are called, MUST be received from your diet. They include what are called the omega-3 and omega-6 groups.

Not eating enough **omega-3** fats—for example, fish, fish oil, walnuts or flax—will create an imbalance with other fats. Flax oil is one of the best sources from which to get your omega-3 fats, and I recommend you consume this liberally.

Omega-3 fatty acids have been shown to help prevent cancer. Grass-fed beef, wild-caught fish and free-range chicken are all very high in omega-3 fats and contain far more omega-3 than their grain-fed, farm-raised and caged counterparts. Apparently there are studies that show that eating red meat causes cancer. I would like to see a study done on the consumption of grass-fed beef versus corn-fed beef. As the ratio of omega-3 in the former is so much higher, my guess is that you would see a significant reduction in cancer among the group eating the grass-fed meat.

Omega-6 foods include sunflower seeds, sesame seeds, pumpkin seeds, evening primrose oil, borage oil, olive oil and olives, almonds, pine nuts, pistachio nuts, Brazil nuts, walnuts, hazelnuts, peanut oil—unprocessed (hard to find)—and avocados. Many of these foods have a combination of both omega-3 and omega-6 fats. Even grass-fed beef and pasture-raised chicken, as well as eggs from pasture-raised chickens, have a combination of omega-3 and omega-6, and grass-fed meats in general have far greater quantities of omega fats than grain-fed animals.

You need a 1:1 ratio of omega-3 and omega-6 fats.

The requirement for these fats (in nut and seed form) should be at least one handful per day. Getting them directly from food is better than using a supplement; however, any form is better than none at all. These essential fats supply the raw material with which to make cell walls and are used as well in the structure of your mitochondria (cellular energy factories). If building a house needs wood, your cells need omega fats, and their presence in the body enables oxygen to travel easily through the cells. There are very credible studies showing that cancer grows in areas of your body where a decrease in oxygen occurs. Essential fatty acid deficiencies are behind this decreased oxygen situation and are also a prime cause of dry skin and hair.

Trans Fats

Also known as trans fatty acids and hydrogenated or partially hydrogenated fats, these are man-made or processed fats, produced by adding hydrogen gas to a liquid fat or oil to make it thicker or more solid. This increases its shelf life, as it is less likely to spoil.

If you are consuming trans fats (margarine, artificial butters, either partially or completely hydrogenated), your liver will be stressed. They are like edible plastic and are very hard on the liver. Acceptable fats to use in place of these are olive oil, flax oil, safflower oil, butter and coconut oil.

The best cooking oils are coconut oil, safflower oil, olive oil and peanut oil. I recommend that you cook with coconut oil, since it has been demonstrated to have a positive effect on metabolism. The other good point about coconut oil is that it doesn't require much of the liver's bile to break it down, which means less stress on the liver. Bile is the detergent that breaks down grease or fatty foods.

Saturated Fats

Saturated fats are found mainly in animal products and also in certain plant foods.

Consuming excessive heavy saturated fats, such as bacon, sausage and overcooked beef, can stress the liver and especially the gallbladder. If a person has a healthy liver, some better-quality saturated fats can help with weight loss. The fats I recommend are coconut oil, butter, avocado, cream, cream cheese, rare steak and hamburger.

Eating more fat can sometimes increase the burning of stored fat.[13] I have had patients finally lose weight when they started increasing fats in their diets—avocados, butter and coconut butter. When the body receives this fat, it activates more fat-dissolving enzymes (lipases—things that break down lipids, or fats); also, fat has the antidote to cholesterol—lecithin. If you restrict fats in the diet, the body compensates by slowing the breakdown of fats; it goes into a holding mode. I have found that when a person who is trying to lose weight and doing everything correctly is still having a hard time, adding more fat can sometimes speed up weight loss.

A rule of thumb is *the worse the liver, the less fat you can tolerate in your diet.* Just go lighter on fats if you notice any bloating. It does take some time for your body to adjust to the digestion of fats. Some people cannot even tolerate too many raw nuts; however, one handful of seeds or nuts would be easily tolerated by most.

The Adrenal and Ovary body types require more fats than the Liver and Thyroid types.

Trigger #5

Skipping Meals and Intermittent Fasting

In the prior edition, I suggested not skipping meals, especially breakfast. I also recommended eating frequent meals (four to five smaller meals throughout the day). Both advices were wrong.

I am constantly adapting my plan to what works best for most people, so I am very willing to be wrong and not hold on to any fixed ideas. The goal is to find what works.

I want to come back to the hormone insulin. I have recently learned of additional insulin triggers that go beyond the sugar-triggering effect. I am not sure how I missed this when I initially studied the data on insulin in Guyton's *Textbook of Medical Physiology*, but here's what I found: Every time you eat, no matter what the food, you trigger insulin to some degree. Thus, you can imagine that eating four to five small meals every day is guaranteed to completely keep you from losing fat—it causes insulin spikes all day long.

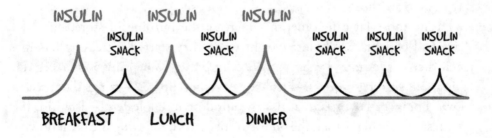

So many people think snacking is healthy. And grazing at night becomes, for some, a habit and a way of life. Whether out of boredom or stress, people have to put things in their mouths constantly. It's the frequent spike in insulin that causes insulin resistance. And if we have four to five spikes of insulin throughout the day, you'll never fix insulin resistance. Your body created a resistance to insulin for a reason—it's trying to tell you to avoid the stuff!

The first target is to eliminate snacking.

There are many ways to do intermittent fasting. I suggest you do it in stages, starting out with three meals, without regard to time, but no snacking in between.

The next stage is to keep your eating in an 8-hour window and fast for 16 hours. If you eat breakfast at 10:00 a.m., then dinner would be at 6:00 p.m., and lunch could be around 2:00 p.m. This gives you 16 hours of fasting and 8 hours of eating.

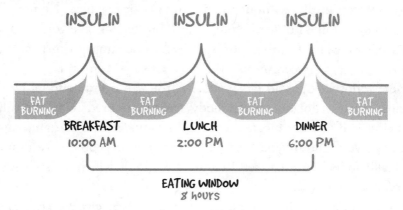

As your body adapts to burning fat, you may want to get into some serious fat burning and do just two meals per day. This involves fasting for 20 hours and eating only in your 4-hour window. Your first meal could be around 12:00 noon and your last meal at 4:00 p.m.

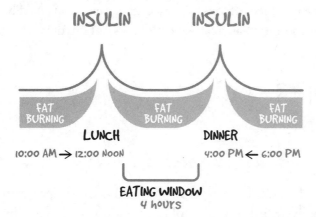

Think about it: If you don't eat, you keep insulin way down. This will greatly reduce the need for a diabetic to have to take drugs that lower blood sugars.

And the "meal" you are eating when you are not eating is your own belly fat. Isn't that the goal?

But how does one go that long without a snack?

There is a secret. . . . Ready?

Adding fat to meals.

This will allow you to go longer without the need to eat frequently. I do not expect you to be starving between meals. In fact, you should feel good between meals, without intense hunger or cravings. It's not a bad thing to have some hunger before a meal, but feeling like you're starving isn't what we want. In other words, if you're not hungry, don't eat; but if you are hungry between meals, add more fat to your meals.

Here's another tip: add fats gradually. You can overdo adding fats and overload your gallbladder. Your body has to get used to it and adjust. Start slowly. If you feel bloated, with right-shoulder pain or right-scapular tightness, you'll know you overdid it. For lots of people, I recommend the Gallbladder Formula (see Resources section), which assists with the digestion of extra fat.

Understanding the dynamic aspects of hormones can give you an advantage in losing weight. For example, when you eat a low-calorie, low-fat bran muffin, insulin is activated, which not only converts the muffin into fat but prevents any burning of stored fat. However, consuming fats, which have higher calories, doesn't have this same effect; in fact, fat doesn't trigger insulin. That is why a tiny piece of low-fat, low-calorie candy can actually prevent the loss of fat much more than a fatty piece of low-carbohydrate cheesecake.

Trigger #6

Gland Destroyers

Alcohol (beer, wine or mixed drinks)

Not only does alcohol trigger insulin and cause weight gain but it also destroys the liver. Just a little alcohol at night can set your liver back for several days. What I mean by setting the liver back is preventing the liver from burning fat. The positive fat-burning effects from foods and exercise can likewise be canceled out by alcohol. You can eat really well and then that small amount of alcohol at dinner can keep you out of fat burning. Alcohol can also trigger the destructive hormone cortisol, since alcohol puts stress on the body. This constant irritation causes inflammation and scarring of the liver, which, in some cases, will not show up on blood tests until it is in the advanced stages.[14] Major scar tissue in the liver is the condition known as cirrhosis. Some people can get away with drinking alcohol merely because their livers and endocrine glands have not yet been destroyed.

Caffeinated Products (coffee, soda, tea and chocolate)

Caffeine stimulates and weakens the adrenal glands and liver and also irritates the gallbladder. It increases cortisol, which can put fat into and around the abdominal organs. If the adrenals are in very bad shape, I don't recommend coming off caffeine too quickly, as lethargy and other withdrawal symptoms can last up to three days, though in most cases it's one to two days. I would recommend cutting down to one small cup of coffee in the morning and then gradually lessening the amount over a two-week period until it's eliminated altogether. It has been shown that drinking two and a half cups of coffee can more than double the stress hormone adrenaline.[15] Even though adrenaline is a fat-burning hormone, the increased cortisol counters this effect. Cortisol tends to stay in the bloodstream much longer—up to eight hours. A sick liver will not be able to rid itself of cortisol very well, causing this hormone to stay in the body even longer. Increasing cortisol lowers growth hormone (fat-burning and anti-aging); and because cortisol is being released, excess stored sugar is being released, causing insulin to convert it to fat around the stomach.

The liver is forced to detoxify the caffeine from coffee; this puts more strain on the liver. I recommend switching to Roma (a coffee-like beverage) or organic water-processed decaf coffee, as commercial decaffeinated coffees can contain toxic chemicals used in removing the caffeine.

Appetite suppressants are stimulants, which in many cases contain caffeine. Caffeine is even sold in pill form at the gas station to help truck drivers stay awake. Herbal stimulants, which do not contain caffeine, can have the ability to stimulate and burn out your glands—including ma huang (ephedra), guarana, gotu kola and kava.

Sodas, tea and chocolate also contain caffeine and so have the same effect. Caffeine, in addition, depletes calcium and B vitamins from the body. Other than that, it is totally fine! Sparkling water is a good substitute. Herb tea (decaffeinated) is likewise a good alternative. Green tea is another beneficial way to transition because, despite having some caffeine, it has an anti-caffeine effect; but here again, naturally decaffeinated green tea would be the better choice.

Drugs

Recreational drugs and medications of all kinds have side effects on the glands, especially the liver. Psychiatric drugs deplete hormones and also make it hard to lose weight. Hormone-replacement hormones and birth-control pills both contain estrogen, which is a fattening hormone. Prednisone is an anti-inflammatory steroid (adrenal hormone), which is also fattening. Insulin is a fat-making hormone. Anti-cholesterol and blood pressure medications have side effects on the liver as well. Diuretics deplete minerals, which can affect the adrenal glands. Antibiotics kill your friendly bacteria, putting stress on your liver because of stress on digestion. These chemicals and others can be big barriers to losing weight. However, I'm not suggesting you come off your medication without the advice of a competent medical doctor.

Detoxification (*toxin* meaning "poison," + *de-*, "to remove")

The liver is the main organ that is supposed to eliminate these chemicals, in two phases. In the first phase the liver tries to neutralize toxins. In the second phase it will try to convert the neutralized toxins into less harmful particles, which can be eliminated through the bladder and bowel.

The following are examples of substances handled by the liver in phase I and II detoxification: drugs, steroids, heavy metals, fertilizers, solvents, environmental estrogens, food additives and dyes, sulfites added in salads you buy in the grocery store (salad bars), sulfites in wines, nitrates in deli meats, synthetic perfumes and makeup absorbed through the skin, alcohol, antibiotics, cigarette smoke, protein waste from high-protein diets, pesticides, exhaust fumes, charcoal-grilled meats, paint fumes, viruses, bacteria, yeast, candida, fungus and molds. Your own excess hormones are also either deactivated or recycled within your liver.

There are specific foods that the liver needs in the process of detoxification. These foods include the cruciferous vegetable family: cabbage, broccoli, Brussels sprouts, kale, radish and collard greens. However, beets and their leaves are extra powerful in the deactivation of estrogens. I have found that patients who include beets in their diets each day (raw, grated, cut up on salads) start noticing increased sex drive and improved lean muscle mass. Their blood pressure also seems to be lower. I believe some of these effects are due to decreased estrogen, allowing testosterone to come to its normal level, along with the massive amounts of potassium in beet tops (leaves), which helps to lower blood pressure. Just one cup of beet tops contains 1,300 milligrams of potassium. Additionally, beets and beet leaves allow for the clearing of the stress hormones cortisol and adrenaline, which is great for people who have anxiety, constipation or sleep problems. I add beet leaves to my kale shake.

Growth Hormones

The animals whose products we eat (meats, milk, cheese), including farm-raised fish, are fed growth hormones. Some are estrogens and some are a type of growth hormone. It is my personal opinion that these hormones have greatly damaged our endocrine glands.

Endocrine Disruptors

As covered previously, pesticides, insecticides, heavy metals, etc., all can mimic estrogen within your glands. These chemicals are on the golf course, in the schools, in restaurants, in your garden, and on your vegetables unless you eat organic. Being exposed to DDT as children, or consuming fruits that have been sprayed with DDT and shipped in from third-world countries, has damaging effects on us. Vaccines also have heavy metals and formaldehyde in them. The amalgam (mercury) in our teeth and the mercury in tuna can affect our hormones. I would recommend switching to organic, hormone-free foods as much as possible (at least 50 percent).

Food and Cosmetic Chemicals

Food preservatives, food dyes, synthetic sugars (dextrose), hydrogenated oils, and even things like synthetic vanilla flavoring all have a bad effect on our glands. Also, skin creams, makeup, shampoos and perfumes can easily absorb through the skin and end up in your liver. Did you know if you rub some garlic or an onion onto the bottom of your foot that within 10 minutes you'll be able to taste garlic or onion? Creams, lotions and cosmetics do absorb through your skin and, through the bloodstream, travel to the liver. Your skin is an indicator of the health of your liver. It is ironic that people are trying to make their skin look better through cosmetics, when these are the very things that are worsening their skin.

Consuming Food without Enzymes

Enzymes are proteins that do ALL the work of the body. Without enzymes, body reactions would take years to occur. Enzymes not only help you digest but help rid your liver of toxic chemicals, stop inflammation, reduce blood pressure and cholesterol, regulate temperature, make hormones, and build body tissues such as hair, nails and skin. Enzymes are the workhorses of the body, and when you consume food without enzymes, you are depleting your enzyme reserve.

You could look at the body as an enzyme bank or reserve. Let's say you ate some food without the enzymes to break down fat (called lipases); your body would then have to release its own lipase reserve. Over time, you can exhaust this supply, creating strain on the glands and organs. Animals that were fed roasted nuts, for example, developed enlarged pancreases, since the pancreas is the key organ to produce and release enzymes. In other words, consuming cooked, steamed, pasteurized, roasted, processed or refined foods forces your body to deplete its enzyme bank, leaving you with degenerative disease.

The first area to repair in an enzyme-depleted body is the glands. This is why we start you out with lots of raw, enzyme-rich foods.

Trigger #7

Water Retainers

A huge hidden source of being overweight is water weight.

When people come into our clinic weighing 250 to 350 pounds with normal or just barely over the normal amounts of body fat, it startles them to realize that most of their weight is water weight.

For example, a 30-year-old male weighing in at 264 pounds had body fat of 24.6 percent. Normal body fat for his age and height is 24.6 percent. In other words, his body fat percentage was perfect, yet his belly was huge. I found out he was loading up his body with massive quantities of hidden fluid retainers. He couldn't believe it when I told him he was not fat.

Another 40-year-old patient weighing in at 350 pounds had 35.7 percent body fat. His normal should have been 26.5 percent. That's only 9.2 percent above normal—not bad. His doctor had told him previously to drink two and a half gallons of water per day to flush out his fat. I put him on the eating plan and he began losing weight steadily every week and was feeling great.

Monosodium glutamate is the big culprit in causing water retention, and it can be hidden under a variety of names: modified food starch, autolyzed yeast, hydrolyzed protein, hydrolyzed vegetable protein, carrageenan, glutamic acid and yeast extract. MSG is also present in most protein isolates (soy isolates, whey isolates, etc.). Many Chinese restaurants will tell you they don't add MSG, yet it's in their sauces under other names. I can taste if food has MSG—it tastes just a bit too good and I can keep eating more than usual; but the next day my finger joints ache and feel puffy.

Many boxed foods, canned foods, gravies, sauces, mixes, TV dinners, lunch foods, hot dogs and condiments have either MSG or lots of chemicals or preservatives that cause water retention. Eating at restaurants gives you a good dose of MSG. It's a difficult substance to avoid. When dining out, keep away from breaded foods and foods with creamy sauces. Eat whole foods with just a few spices. If it is unavoidable, counter the sodium with lots of leafy greens or vegetables, which are high in potassium.

When shopping, make sure you read the labels, especially for the sodium amounts, as you will find that most packaged and processed foods contain mega sodium. They don't list potassium unfortunately, which is the opposing mineral. I have found a product called Kettle Chips to have higher potassium than sodium. However, potato is a starch and will not help you lose weight.

An additional note on MSG: In animal studies, MSG has been shown to triple the output of insulin. Insulin is not only the major fat-making hormone, it is the main preventer of fat burning. In the presence of insulin, your body can NOT burn fat.

Artificial sweeteners, which are in thousands of foods, cause water retention, especially the diet sodas that so many people drink. These include aspartame, saccharin and acesulfame K. Sugar alcohols, such as erythritol, xylitol or mannitol, are another type of artificial sweetener. The two sugar alcohols that I recommend are xylitol and erythritol. The key is making sure they are non-GMO. Some people might also feel that they add bloating or gas or create a laxative effect.

Excess sodium causes increased water retention and decreases potassium. The adrenal hormones are affected indirectly when this mineral imbalance is created.

A major hidden source of potassium-depleting, sodium-retaining foods is refined sugars and carbohydrates. In order to digest sugar, potassium is required. And because potassium is not normally present in white sugar or white flour, you end up using your potassium reserves. Since the cell is where most of the potassium is located, a depletion of this mineral will cause dehydration in the cell with fluid retention outside the cell. This is why you feel puffy and have ankle swelling after eating something sweet, and why consuming sweets makes you thirsty. It is also why you can gain and lose five pounds in a day or gain five pounds overnight. It isn't fat; it's water, which comes with the increased sodium.

Alcohol causes water retention as well.

It would be a good idea to take a look at how many water retainers you are exposed to on a weekly basis and compare this to how many high-potassium foods you eat.

Trigger #8

Exercise

A very interesting yet rarely understood fact of exercise is that the calories burned during exercise are very few. For example, it would take one hour of golfing (walking without a cart) to burn several teaspoons of Thousand Island dressing. However, the delayed fat-burning effects from this exercise are quite significant. You experience most of the fat burning 14 to 48 hours after the exercise—BUT only if certain things are in place. Burning this fat depends on what you eat during this time, how much stress you experience, whether you have pain or not, how much you sleep, and if you are avoiding sugar completely. This is why you don't have to pay too much attention to calories, only to hormones; if you do this, you'll be much more successful.

Eating carbohydrates before, during or after you exercise will prevent the fat-burning effects.[16]

You have probably been told, "Eat everything in moderation," right? This is bad advice. Eating sugar even in small amounts will keep you out of fat burning. Eat protein at least 75 minutes before exercising—but don't stuff yourself. It is okay to eat protein after the exercise as well.[17] Exercise inhibits the fat-making and fat-storing hormone insulin.[18]

Intense anaerobic (higher-pulse-rate or resistance-type) exercise triggers several fat-burning hormones—growth hormone, testosterone, adrenaline and glucagon.[19] However, if the adrenal glands are fatigued or exhausted, intense exercise can prevent weight loss because the stress glands are being overtaxed. If your adrenals are stressed, only do light aerobics (low-pulse-rate endurance-type), if any at all, until you get your energy back and your sleep is improved.

Anaerobic exercise: Higher-pulse-rate (greater than 145 beats per minute), intense resistance-type.

Aerobic exercise: Low-pulse-rate (less than 130 beats per minute) endurance-type.

It's true that the low-pulse-rate (aerobic) exercise burns fat during the time you are doing it, but only after the first 20 to 30 minutes. So if you exercise 40 minutes per day, this is only 10 minutes of fat burning—very insignificant. On the other hand, the intense, high-pulse-rate (anaerobic) exercise does not burn fat during the exercise but triggers fat-burning hormones 14 to 48 hours later.

During the exercise, you are tearing down muscle tissue and causing cortisol to help break down muscle. Then the growth hormone comes in to repair and rebuild it. The fat-burning benefits occur in the rest period when the body is building back up. There is more on this in chapter 17, "Exercising for Your Body Type."

Trigger #9

Stress

Stress can severely affect your weight.

Stress increases the hormone cortisol, which can lead to fat being deposited in and around the abdomen.[20] This is because the adrenal hormone releases a good supply of stored sugar (from both liver and muscles) into the bloodstream, causing insulin to change it into fat.

Types of stress could be contact with poison ivy, receiving a burn or an injury, loss of a loved one, fighting with your spouse, dealing with an angry employer, constipation, not sleeping, getting a hot flash, watching the news (usually negative), reading the newspaper (death, scandal, hurricanes) or hanging out with negative people, as well as having pain or inflammation in your body. If you have pain, cortisol is raised. Pain can prevent weight loss because the hormone cortisol raises sugar and blocks fat from being burned.

I have developed amazing do-it-yourself acupressure techniques, using a massage tool that mimics my own hand. I originally designed it to work on myself. You'll learn more about this tool later. The techniques release the accumulated stress in your body. I have isolated areas on the body that store most of your stress; by releasing it, you can help your body get into a wonderful deep and restful sleep.

Exercise can reduce stress; however, exercise can also increase stress on the body because it increases cortisol. The goal is to exercise in a way so as to not raise cortisol too much. This would mean keeping your pulse rate low during exercise. Weight training is resistance-type exercise and increases cortisol unless you do fewer repetitions and rest between them. You also would not want to exercise over soreness.

A few anti-stress activities include walking, hiking, slow endurance-type exercise, being outside, working around the yard, avoiding the computer screen, and avoiding reading the newspaper or watching the five o'clock TV news station. Try reading a book before bed instead of watching TV.

Trigger #10

Sleep

The fat-burning growth hormone is active throughout the night while you sleep; however, it increases during the first two hours of deep sleep, especially between midnight and 4:00 a.m.[21] Omitting this sleep can prevent the fat-burning effect. In other words, the reason why you burn more fat during sleep is because the fat-burning growth hormone spikes during deep sleep cycles. It's difficult to catch up on that important sleep if you miss this time period.

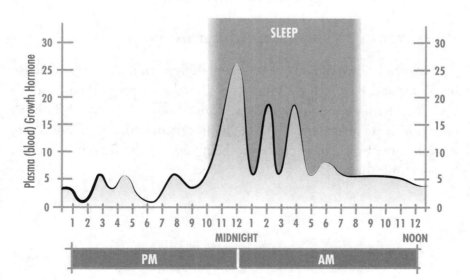

CIRCADIAN RHYTHM AND GROWTH HORMONE

When you sleep, you typically go through four 90-minute cycles of light and deep sleep. Light sleep is REM (rapid eye movement) sleep, which is very active, producing lots of dreaming that you can remember. Delta-wave sleep is the deepest, in which you can dream but usually can't remember the dreams. Not getting quality sleep or getting inadequate sleep (less than seven hours) can prevent fat burning. You burn fat in the deeper sleep cycles, which could be a huge barrier for many people. You can't induce a deep rejuvenating sleep artificially through medication and expect to get these fat-burning effects; it has to be real natural sleep.

The delayed fat-burning effects of exercise can be prevented if you are not sleeping or if you eat sugar before, during or after exercise. If cortisol (stress hormone) is too high, not only will deep rejuvenating sleep be prevented[22]—which will affect the fat-burning growth hormone—but fat will be directed to and stored in the belly.

Eating before Bed

Eating or drinking refined sugars before going to bed (for example, orange juice) can nullify growth hormone's fat-burning effects as well as keep insulin high enough to prevent any fat release.[23] This includes a glass of wine. Four sticks of celery are a better snack before bed. Celery contains active compounds called pthalides, which relax the muscles of the arteries and also reduce adrenal (stress) hormones.

Nutritional Supplementation and Sleep

Sleep can be interrupted due to several things: hot flashes, an overactive bladder, pain, restless legs, and so on. But the most common cause is just body tension and stress. It's as if your body's "on" switch is stuck on. This is an overactive fight-or-flight system (adrenals). For sleep, there is something I have created to help you; see the Resources section for more information.

10

Fat-Burning Strategies

Before we get into the eating plan, you need to understand several key principles. Very few people know how to burn fat as their main fuel. I need to show you how to do this.

The worst approach is to search online and just start trying different things. Or worse yet, accept some advice from a neighbor: "Hey, why don't you try . . . ?" Too many people simply keep guessing.

Let me take you behind the scenes and give you a bit of physiology in understandable terms.

Losing weight is a very unnatural thing. Your body does not like to lose anything because that goes against its purpose of surviving. In fact it fights losing weight by slowing metabolism. Fat loss is an anti-survival activity, since fat to the body is stored survival fuel. Yes, diets slow one's metabolism—this is why.

The ONLY way to lose weight without slowing the metabolism is to increase health. Unfortunately, the way some people define *health* is inaccurate: "I am healthy because all my symptoms are being managed by my prescription drugs." So let's first define health.

> HEALTH is a condition of high energy, excellent sleep, great vitality, no cravings, excellent digestion, no inflammation, high tolerance for stress, and great memory. Health occurs when all the body's organs and glands are working together.

Now let's look at how to create a healthy metabolism and fix the key hormones that control it.

There are two main fuel sources involved in metabolism:

- Fat

- Sugar (glucose)

What determines which one is burned (or metabolized) is a hormone called INSULIN. It is the most important switch that affects your body's fat burning.

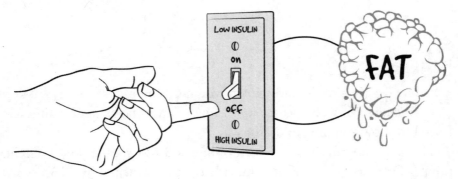

What Is Insulin?

Insulin is associated with diabetes because it controls blood sugars. It's a hormone made by the pancreas and it gets triggered by sugar (carbs). It lowers sugars in your blood after meals. If you have an unhealthy insulin problem, as in diabetes, insulin doesn't do its job of lowering sugars, and blood sugars go screaming high. Insulin lowers blood sugar!

Insulin deals with sugar in three ways:

1. Causes cells to absorb sugar fuel

2. Converts sugar to stored sugar (glycogen)

3. Converts sugar to fat and cholesterol

So the question is, what diet should you be on? And the answer is you should be on the one that fixes this broken switch called insulin. By getting insulin healthy again, not only will you burn fat and restore metabolism, but you'll also begin to solve lots of other problems as well.

This is not theory but a fundamental fact that can be learned from one of the world's most credible physiology texts, Guyton's *Textbook of Medical Physiology*, which clearly explains two things: (1) in the absence of insulin, the body will use fat exclusively; and (2) in the presence of insulin, all aspects of fat burning are shut off.

Okay, now that we've gotten that out of the way, we need to know HOW to lower insulin, right?

Isn't it a matter of cutting out the sugars?

Partially.

If you only cut out the sugars, you can improve things by 50 percent.

For the other 50 percent of the strategy, let's go back to Guyton and see what he says.

> "Formerly, it was believed that insulin secretion is controlled almost entirely by the blood glucose concentration. In addition to excess glucose stimulating insulin secretion, many of the amino acids have a similar effect."
>
> —*Textbook of Medical Physiology,* page 930

Amino acids are proteins, and these can trigger insulin. Interesting. Guyton goes on to say that when you consume glucose with protein, you can greatly accentuate or double insulin levels. So hold off on the burger, fries and coke or the hamburger and bun for right now, okay?

The other point he makes is that excess protein can spike insulin too. So avoid the Texas-style steaks (18 ounces!) as well. I know this will be hard, but do your best.

Although we have discussed it a bit in previous chapters, I want to spend time on this next trigger and really hit it home due to its importance.

There is ONE more important point Dr. Guyton makes about insulin triggers.

> "Gastrointestinal hormones almost double the rate of insulin secretion following an average meal."
>
> —*Textbook of Medical Physiology,* page 930

Every time you eat, you trigger insulin. This is why snacks between meals are bad for weight loss. This is also why intermittent fasting is very healthy to heal insulin.

Intermittent Fasting

As covered in chapter 9, under Trigger #5, I am suggesting you start out with a simple version of intermittent fasting: no snacks between meals. Here's why.

If you snack between meals, you trigger some insulin. The way insulin got messed up in the first place was higher levels of sustained insulin being triggered over time. Listen, if you exercised all day long and never gave yourself a chance to recover or rest, what would happen? In this case, you never give your insulin a chance to recover from the sustained insulin outflow.

We need to fix the insulin problem by keeping it low between meals. This way we can switch to fat burning between meals and especially at night. So, only three meals with no snacking in between.

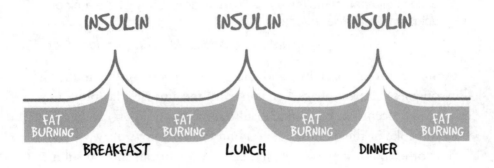

And if you are not hungry in the morning, don't eat! It's okay to have two meals per day.

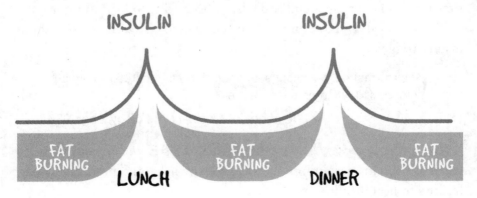

Eating six small meals per day to stimulate your metabolism is a big myth and very bad advice, unless you're trying to gain weight—and do it in an unhealthy way.

If you skip a meal, your body will turn your belly fat into a meal. Isn't this the point, the goal, to use your fat as fuel? Then we need to keep insulin down.

Sustained eating with snacks destroys insulin regulation.

Summary on insulin triggers:

- Avoid sugar.
- Avoid eating protein and sugar together.
- Avoid excess protein.
- Avoid snacking.

You may have heard of the glycemic index. If not, the glycemic index is the scale of how fast a food turns into glucose (blood sugar). White bread is a lot higher on the scale than celery, for example—although both are carbs.

But I'll bet you have not heard of the insulin index, have you? The insulin index measures all the non-carbohydrate triggers of insulin.

When you go to the doctor, he will test the sugar in your blood, right? But does he ever test insulin levels? Testing fasting insulin levels would give some deeper insights.

Research on the insulin index gives us a scale that ranges from things that barely trigger insulin to things that majorly trigger insulin.

Certain types of protein trigger insulin more than others. Apparently whey protein, egg whites or other low-fat, lean proteins can spike insulin way more than whole-fat protein foods. If we combine the egg yolk with the egg white and eat it like Mother Nature intended, insulin response is much lower.

This goes against everything we have been taught. People have been focusing on low-fat *everything*.

I am not telling you to completely avoid everything that triggers insulin, because protein can also stimulate your metabolism, in the right amounts. And we need some protein to replace what our bodies are made from. (Interestingly, no part of the body is made of carbohydrate, and there are no essential carbs; only essential fatty acids and essential amino acids—proteins.)

However, if we add sugar to protein, we get an amplified, exaggerated insulin spike. And I am talking hamburger and bun, hot dog and ketchup, burger and coke, burger and fries.

But the most fascinating thing about the insulin index is dietary fats. Pure fats hardly trigger insulin at all.

Wow!

In fact, fat can slow the effects of insulin.

Check this out:

Fat-free pretzels rate 81 percent—extremely high—yet bacon is only 9 percent (very low) on the insulin index.

Low-fat yogurt rates 76 percent, and if we add sugar and sweeten it, the rating goes up to 115 percent.

Egg whites rate 55 percent, but egg yolks are only 15 percent; so if we combine them, we get 21 percent.

What does all this mean? It means that for years we've been focused on the wrong villain. Fat is not the bad guy. Low-fat and lean proteins actually trigger insulin more than whole-fat proteins.

Insulin Index

2% Butter	11% Tahini butter (sesame seed)
3% Olives/Olive oil	11% Pork
3% Coconut oil	11% Peanut butter
3% Flax oil	12% Cod fish
4% Heavy cream	12% Duck
5% Pecans	13% Peanuts
5% Macadamia nuts	13% Pork sausage
6% Avocado	14% Pumpkin
7% Coconut meat	14% Almonds
8% Cream cheese	15% Cheddar cheese
8% Sour cream	15% Sunflower seeds
9% Bacon	15% Chia seeds
9% Walnuts	15% Egg yolk
9% Pine nuts	16% Blue cheese
10% Pepperoni	19% Pistachios

20% Coleslaw
21% Swiss cheese
21% Whole egg
23% Turkey
24% All-Bran
24% Chicken
25% Low-fat cream cheese
29% Pasta
40% Whole milk
43% Low-fat swiss cheese
47% Berries
51% Beef
54% Popcorn
55% Egg whites
59% Scallops

59% Fish
61% Potato chips
62% Brown rice
75% Apple
76% Low-fat yogurt
81% Fat-free pretzel
84% Banana
87% Crackers
96% Whole-wheat bread
100% White bread
100% Baked beans
115% Sweetened yogurt
121% Potatoes
160% Jelly beans

Is there anything else?

Yes, there is one more big one. Cortisol—the stress hormone!

An overactive adrenal pumping out excessive cortisol causes your body to release or make new sugar. In other words, stress spikes insulin. This explains why people gain weight after a stress event. I mean, look at the side effect of the adrenal-stress-hormone medication cortisone shots (prednisone). One side effect is diabetes. Why? Because cortisol releases a ton of sugar, and sugar triggers insulin.

Insulin Resistance

The great majority of people with belly fat have a condition called *insulin resistance*. It's a prediabetic situation where the body's cells are rejecting insulin or blocking it. The cells sense low insulin, so they will trigger the pancreas to make a lot more—four to five times more. As a result, insulin is lower in some places (cells, brain, muscles, blood, etc.) yet higher in other places in the body. It's very similar to talking to someone with ear plugs, who doesn't hear you until you start shouting. The feedback circuitry for insulin "doesn't hear" the insulin, so a signal is sent back to the pancreas telling it to make more.

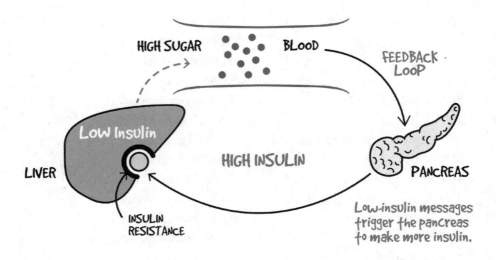

People with insulin resistance have four to five times more insulin in their bodies even when they are fasting.

These are the symptoms of insulin resistance:

- Cravings for sweets
- Not satisfied after eating
- Can't go long without hunger
- Mood improves with eating
- Tired after lunch (or meals)
- Impaired eyesight
- Worsened memory
- Belly fat
- Liver fat
- Fatigue
- Irritability
- High blood pressure
- Fluid retention
- Frequent urination at night
- PCOS (polycystic ovarian syndrome)

Insulin resistance is what causes your weight to plateau at a certain level. Handling insulin resistance is the only way I know to fix a stuck metabolism.

Polycystic Ovarian Syndrome

The higher levels of insulin lead to the creation of more androgens (male hormones), causing PCOS (polycystic ovarian syndrome) in females; this in turn can result in weight gain, insulin resistance, facial hair and acne. It's interesting: if you research PCOS, you will always find insulin resistance as a symptom; but PCOS and insulin resistance are only loosely associated by most sources. What they don't realize is that insulin resistance is *causing* PCOS. This is why PCOS disappears when insulin resistance disappears; try it and you'll see for yourself.

High Blood Pressure

One of the side effects of insulin resistance is high blood pressure. This is due to a potassium deficiency. You see, insulin controls the intake of potassium into your cells. Potassium is the key mineral that relaxes the arteries, keeps them elastic, prevents sodium from causing excess fluid, and keeps the blood pressure low. People who are salt sensitive are really potassium deficient. Compounding this problem by adding a diuretic further depletes potassium, the very thing that could correct this sensitivity.

Adding a good amount of vegetables to your eating plan raises potassium and lessens the need for insulin, thus lowering its resistance.

What Spikes Insulin

1. Sugar and hidden sugars
2. Concentrated low-fat or lean protein
3. Large amounts of protein eaten in a meal
4. Combining protein with sugar
5. MSG and hidden MSG (modified food starch)
6. Frequent meals (snacks)
7. Stress (cortisol)
8. The insulin drug (when you are a diabetic)

Corrective Actions

As you correct your eating based on the following tips, your cravings will go down close to zero, and you will be satisfied after meals. You will be clearing up the symptoms of insulin resistance.

Keep Your Sugar at Zero

Start reading labels, focusing mostly on sugar grams. You must avoid consuming sugar and hidden sugars. But anytime we take something away, people want it more, right? No worries; I have an entire section on substitute foods and some delicious dessert recipes in chapters 13 and 18.

Add More Fat

The point I am making about fat is that you do not want to go toward low-fat or lean anything. However, I am not saying eat excessive amounts. You want to eat enough fat per meal to be able to go to the next meal without too much hunger. Not having enough fat will make it impossible to do intermittent fasting. This recommended fat includes foods low on the insulin index: butter, olives, bacon, heavy cream, and peanut or almond butter. The key is to be able to go from one meal to the next without intense hunger and cravings. Adjust your fats so you are able to do this. Some people need a bit more than others, but once you hit the sweet spot, maybe by adding more bacon or Brie cheese to a meal, then it becomes easier. It is not that fat is causing the weight loss; instead it's the fact that fat is allowing you to go longer without eating and raising your insulin.

No Snacking

Even if your snacks are healthy, eating in general will raise insulin a little. Look at this as similar to exercise. The benefits of exercise are in the recovery phase, after you stop exercising. It's the same with eating. When you don't eat between meals, your body switches to fat burning and it's eating your fat—that's the meal we want your body to focus on. The aim is not to lower your calories and graze through the day. Eat healthily but less frequently so the fat-burning switch can be active again, and only consume your fats with a meal.

Additional Tips

Apple Cider Vinegar

I recommend consuming apple cider vinegar in your water each day. It is an amazing way to reactivate your insulin receptors and make glucose absorbable. Taking apple cider vinegar can decrease your need for insulin, thereby improving any blood sugar problem.

Drinking cider vinegar in your water will also help dissolve fat around your liver. I would take 1 tablespoon with a glass of water and drink it with each meal. I also add 1 tablespoon of lemon juice. Lemon is a great way to keep kidney stones from occurring. This drink has two benefits: it will acidify your stomach to improve digestion and it will improve your insulin situation.

Fermented foods like pickles and sauerkraut are also good for improving insulin resistance.

Exercise

Exercise is another great action to improve insulin resistance and speed up metabolism. The secret is to exercise according to your body type. If you are an Adrenal type and you do too much—if you overtrain—you will slow your weight loss down, because of the spike caused by excess stress (cortisol). Adrenal types need long walks or low-intensity exercise, like Pilates. On the other hand, if the adrenals are strong, then add interval training or higher-intensity exercise.

The best way to know what exercise is right for you is to do it and observe how you react to it. If you feel terrible afterwards and can't sleep, and even gain weight, then you know to only walk for now. But despite being an Adrenal type, over time you need to pick up the pace and gradually increase your exercise and intensity. You're not going to be an Adrenal type forever.

If you exercise and become extremely hungry, then we know that your body is only in sugar-burning mode and can't switch to fat burning easily yet. In this case, cut down the exercise. If you exercise and it reduces your hunger, then you can increase the intensity, as your body is burning fat.

You'll learn more on this subject in chapter 17, "Exercising for Your Body Type."

Potassium

Potassium is one of those minerals that is needed in large quantities: over 4,500 milligrams per day. Potassium is necessary for storing sugar as glycogen. (Glycogen is stored sugar.) Having more stored sugar will allow you to go longer without eating, whereas not having enough stored sugar forces your body to have to eat frequently. Therefore, adding more potassium to the diet reduces the need for insulin, thus improving blood sugars. Almost all diabetics are low in potassium.

You actually need 4,700 milligrams of potassium per day. How much food is this equivalent to? You would have to consume 15 bananas or 5 avocados or 7 to 10 cups of certain vegetables each day to get this much potassium. Avocados are very high in potassium, but beet leaves are the highest. Bananas only provide 300 milligrams per banana, and they are too sweet to eat more than 10 a day.

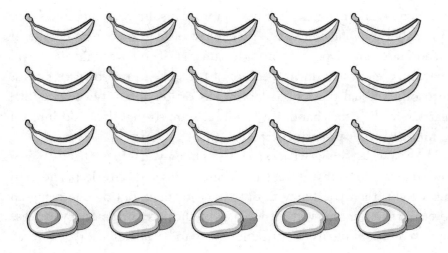

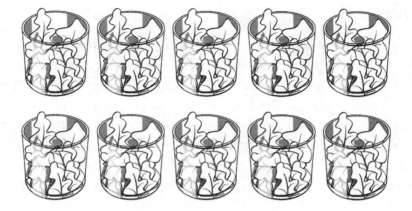

Potassium pills (which I don't advise) only come in 99 milligram tablets. You would have to consume 47 pills a day—not recommended. When we eat the required amount of vegetables, we get ALL our nutrients, not just potassium. Personally, I like to add the food that contains the highest amount of potassium, beet leaves, to my kale shake.

But salads (with mixed greens, including beet tops) have roughly 470–500 milligrams of potassium per cup. I recommend eating two large salads (with mixed veggies) per day to satisfy your potassium requirements. A cup of salad is just a loose handful, not super condensed or pressed into the cup. A bag of salad from your grocery store is between 7 and 8 ounces. One ounce equals one cup.

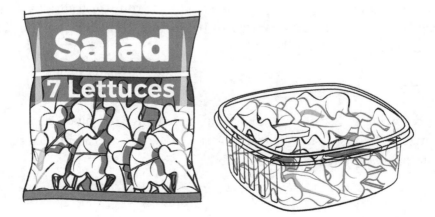

THESE ARE EXAMPLES OF 7 TO 8 CUPS OF SALAD

Vitamin B1

Diabetics are always extremely deficient in B1. Vitamin B1 is needed in your cells for glucose control. In fact, it's the lack of B1 that eventually destroys the nerves in your feet and hands (peripheral neuropathy). And you become deficient in B1 when you eat sugar and refined carbohydrates. That's why you see enriched breads and flours—they add B vitamins. Of course, they add synthetic vitamins.

Vitamin B1 can act as a natural insulin helper, decreasing the need for insulin and thus improving a problem with blood sugars. B1 also helps to prevent an over-acidic condition in diabetes (ketoacidosis or lactic acidosis). The best source of B vitamins is nutritional yeast; take one teaspoon per day in your shakes or mix it with almond butter.

Sleep

Sleep also improves your insulin levels and decreases the stress hormone cortisol. Ask any diabetic what happens to their blood sugar level when they can't sleep or they are in stress, and you'll find out that it worsens things. But we have two scenarios: The first is not being able to sleep, in which case you need to go to chapter 16, "Ridding Your Body of Stress," and use the acupressure techniques for better sleep, or use my Sleep Aid (see Resources section). The next scenario is just not allowing yourself to get enough sleep. Hey, there are a lot of great TV programs late at night, right? If you can get eight-plus hours of sleep, you will really speed up your progress. Make sure you go to bed before 11:00 p.m. so you can work with your natural sleep cycles.

Stress

Reducing stress will be a huge factor in helping your blood sugars. As you have just read, stress releases cortisol, which releases additional sugar into the system. More on this in a bit.

Medications

Unfortunately many of us are using medications that are indirectly worsening our insulin levels. Over time when you improve your health, the need for medication will go down; your doctor hopefully doesn't have the fixed idea that everyone needs to be on meds for the rest of their lives. There are doctors who have the idea that even if your blood values are normal, you need meds as a preventive. That would be great . . . IF those meds didn't have so many side effects. Use your new way of eating as your preventative action.

Medications that worsen insulin:

1. Insulin

2. Cortisol (prednisone, cortisone shots and steroids)

3. High blood pressure meds (diuretics especially)

4. Psychiatric drugs (anti-depressive and anti-anxiety)

And many more; there are over 390 drugs that worsen insulin.*

* *Source:* Diabetes in Control (2016).

11

Step ONE: Basic Eating Plan

In the last edition of this book, each person doing this program started with the Liver Enhancement and then was directed to choose and follow a specific body type. This caused lots of complexities because many people have a mixed body type.

Since then I have greatly simplified things. I have isolated ONE basic eating plan for all four body types. From that point, things can be deleted, added or tweaked—based on how you respond to the basic plan and based on other symptoms that relate to determining your potential body type. For example: If you have an Ovary body type, we need to add foods to lower estrogen. If you have a Liver body type, then you need specific foods to improve liver function and even reduce a fatty liver. And for an Adrenal body type, you need to eat foods that reduce stress. Doing it this way will help keep it simple for you.

The goal is to get your metabolism healthy so it can burn the fat off and keep it off. The bigger goal is to not be one of the four body types!

Is this the ketosis diet?

The answer is, not exactly.

> *Ketosis* is a condition where your body is running on ketones, the byproduct of fat. Ketosis diets involve severely reduced carbohydrates so that your body can switch to fat burning. Ketones are the byproduct of fat burning.

The ketosis diet requires you to consume a good amount of fat. And believe me, I am not against eating fat at all, and I will even say it's not an unhealthy thing to do. However, most people reading this book have a slow metabolism, and when they do the ketosis diet, they end up burning the dietary fat they are eating more than their own fat. And more importantly, if ketosis is done incorrectly, you can end up with a fattier liver.

In this plan we're not going to avoid fat, and we're not going to add tons of fat in the diet either. We have to ensure you get your nutrients; and yes, I am talking vegetables. However, if you're under 25 and skinny, with a fast metabolism (and if so, I'm not sure why you are reading this anyway), you can increase your fats without a problem.

Overall Summary

If you are not hungry in the morning, then avoid eating. It's totally okay to eat two meals a day.

If you are hungry, here's what I suggest you eat. Your breakfast is going to be mainly moderate protein and some fat, but no sugary *anything* (toast, cereal, juice, etc.). If you are a coffee drinker, try to keep it to one small cup in the morning. If you use cream, use either grass-fed or organic. If you normally use sugar in your coffee, use xylitol sweetener instead.

Your lunch and dinner will be a combination of vegetables or salad and non-lean protein (another way of saying fatty protein). You will be adding fat, and the amount you add will be based on how hungry you get between meals.

I do not want you to do any snacks between meals, based on the information in the last chapter. We want your body's snacks to be your belly fat. And if you are not hungry, don't eat—that's the rule. This will give your insulin dysfunction a chance to chill out and heal.

So, there are those things you'll be eating and, MORE IMPORTANTLY, those things you'll be avoiding.

The very cool things that you will be able to include in this plan are listed in the Healthy Pleasure Foods section of this book, in chapter 18— including such treats as peanut butter cups, English muffins, cookies, pancakes, granola, chocolate, and even ice cream. Yes, you heard me right. But let's visit this in a few weeks, if you even need to. I wanted to provide you with some healthy pleasure-food recipes so you never feel deprived. But you will find that once your body has gone completely into fat-burning mode, which takes between two and six weeks, your self-control will be higher and your cravings and hunger will be lower.

Strengthening Your Digestive Weaknesses

I'm sure you've heard the saying "It's not what you eat; it's what you digest and absorb that counts." One primary thing I need to mention is your ability to digest. Is it working?

I am talking about these issues:

- Bloating
- Indigestion
- Acid reflux (or GERD; similar thing)
- Constipation
- Irritable bowel syndrome (IBS)

If we want to be healthy and lose weight, then we cannot have any digestion issues. If you are trying to lose weight when you're constipated, or in spite of having a distended abdomen, that just won't cut it. It is true that the eating plan can help with all these symptoms, but sometimes you may need some Digest Formula and Gallbladder Formula, or even friendly bacteria, to replenish what's been missing.

Bloating

If you bloat from the introduction of cruciferous vegetables, then stop eating them. Though they are healthy, bloating will keep you from losing weight. However, if you bloat even without eating these vegetables, then chances are your gallbladder is not releasing enough bile (digestive fluid). In this case, add 1 Gallbladder Formula after each meal (see Resources section). I also recommend using the apple cider vinegar drink with your meals.

Indigestion

Indigestion is a combination of pain or pressure from food sitting in your stomach too long and not digesting. This comes from a lack of hydrochloric acid (stomach acid). It is extremely common, and many people have low stomach acids, especially as they age. I recommend an acidifier supplement just before meals (take 2 to 4). (See Resources section for more information.)

Acid Reflux, Heartburn (or GERD)

The biggest myth about heartburn is that it is a condition of too much acid, when in fact it is not enough acid. The valve at the top of the stomach, which is responsible for keeping the acid in the stomach, is controlled by the stomach acidity. A low stomach-acid pH will keep the valve open, causing acid to regurgitate (back up) into the esophagus.

Normally the stomach acid is supposed to be at a pH between 1 and 3, which is extremely acidic. As we age, eat poorly or take too many antacids, we lose the acid strength, thus weakening the digestion. Powerful protein enzymes are also controlled by this acid. Without having your stomach acid pH at the right level of acidity, your protein digestion and mineral absorption are hindered. I recommend taking an acidifier supplement before each meal. (See Resources section.)

If by chance you have an ulcer or stomach inflammation from long-term acid reflux, you will need to heal your digestive tract with chlorophyll. For this I recommend using my Raw Wheat Grass Juice Powder for a few weeks before starting any acid products (see Resources section for more info). And one good remedy for ulcers is cabbage juice. I always recommend either drinking cabbage juice or consuming cabbage in the form of coleslaw.

Constipation

You may find that your new eating plan resolves your constipation. If not, there are several causes of constipation that may need addressing. The digestive tract is long, and a dysfunction at any part can leave you with incomplete digestion that backs up the plumbing.

If you developed constipation on this program, then most likely your system is not ready for the quantity of cruciferous vegetables, or specifically kale. Simply change your vegetables to items that you know will not cause a problem. You can also steam them or even consume fermented vegetables, like pickles or sauerkraut. Friendly microbes actually live on fiber, but too much vegetable fiber too fast can overwhelm them.

If you already have been experiencing constipation before this program, let's dissect a possible reason. Ask yourself when it started and what occurred just before. Was it after being given antibiotics? If so, then add intestinal flora back in by taking a high-quality probiotic.

Another common cause of constipation is the lack of bile. Bile not only has the function of digesting fat, but it also acts to lubricate the colon. If you are a vegetarian or have been on a low-fat diet, you may be deficient in bile because bile is triggered by saturated fats. If you have additional symptoms of low bile salts—bloating, right-shoulder pain or tightness, burping or belching—then this could be the cause. Take 1 Gallbladder Formula after meals for this situation.

A further reason for constipation is a lack of stomach acid. If you are not digesting food at the stomach level, it can end up in the colon as undigested material. If you have symptoms of low stomach acid, such as indigestion, acid reflux or GERD, stomach pain when you eat, or an inability to digest red meat, then take between 2 and 4 Digest Formula before meals.

Special Note on Your Gallbladder

The liver makes bile and the gallbladder stores it. Bile is often likened to the detergent that breaks down the grease. It starts the process of dissolving fats and then the pancreas secretes enzymes to complete the process. Without bile, fat digestion is incomplete. This can create a fat-soluble-vitamin deficiency, including low levels of vitamins A, E, D and K.

Saturated fats trigger the release of bile. Yes, I know what you're saying: "I thought fat was bad for the gallbladder." But that's only if the fat is severely excessive or if dietary fat is combined with sugar or grains. Vegetarians who eat no animal fat find that after a while they don't release enough bile and many times end up with gallbladder problems or just an inactive gallbladder and very low amounts of bile. This will dry out their hair, skin and eyes. We need the fat for fat-soluble vitamins, which keep the skin, hair and eyes lubricated and perform a myriad of other functions. Fat-soluble vitamins act like hormones in the body.

Bile also prevents, and can even dissolve, gallstones. If you have had your gallbladder removed, it is likely that you are bile deficient.

Irritable Bowel Syndrome (IBS)

Grains are the most common intestinal irritant, among all the things you can eat, but specifically the protein part of grain—the part called gluten. Gluten is the stuff that makes the texture of bread so gooey and delicious. Many clients ask if oatmeal contains gluten. If it's uncontaminated and pure, the answer is no. However, it is a grain and grains tend to turn into sugars, so avoid it for now. Most oatmeal is low in nutrition as well. Chances are that this eating plan will reduce inflammation in your gut because grains are not in the plan. If you still have intestinal irritation, I recommend added chlorophyll from Raw Wheat Grass Juice Powder due to its healing potential.

It will be important to track your eating closely and make notes on how you feel so you can ensure you avoid food allergies as well. One overweight woman came to see me, and I put her on a very basic healthy-eating regimen. She gained ten pounds in one week. Of course she thought this was fat, but it was fluids from food allergies; you could even see the skin around her eyes was swollen, which is an allergy symptom. Apparently she was allergic to eggs, fish, nuts, cheese—and the list went on and on. After we sent her for some allergy tests, we were able to craft a diet that she could eat, and she started losing weight.

Another common remedy used to repair damage to the intestinal tract is L-glutamine. You can get this at the health food store; it works pretty well to heal the lining of the GI (gastrointestinal, or digestive) tract.

General Overview

This basic eating plan is composed of nutrient-dense food that will nourish and heal your metabolism. There will be additional tweaks, as we go through this program, to address your specific body type; however, I want you to start with the basics.

We want to implement an easy-to-do version of intermittent fasting, with three meals and no snacks between. When you feel comfortable with this, you can even try two meals per day if you want to speed things up. Remember: when you are not eating, you're living off your fat reserves.

Here is a very general idea of what you'll eat:

Breakfast	**Lunch**	**Dinner**
Eggs + bacon + avocado	Big salad or vegetable + protein + fat	Big salad or vegetable + protein + fat

Rules

1. Don't eat when you are not hungry.
2. Don't snack between meals.
3. Add and adjust your fats with meals until you can go from one meal to the next comfortably. If you start with too much fat, you can get bloated.
4. Have two to three meals per day.
5. Drink liquids only when thirsty. I recommend adding 1 tablespoon of apple cider vinegar/1 tablespoon of lemon (fresh-squeezed or bottled lemon juice) to a glass of water and drinking it with meals. To sweeten, add a few drops of liquid stevia.
6. Herbal teas (naturally decaffeinated) are acceptable.
7. Use the following sweeteners if needed: stevia, xylitol (non-GMO), erythritol (non-GMO) or coconut glycerin.
8. Keep sugars as close to zero as possible. This includes agave, honey, dextrose, fructose, etc.
9. Avoid foods that turn into sugar fast: grains, potatoes, rice and fruits. If your metabolism is not too slow, you may be able to get away with a small quantity of berries in your kale shake.

Other Examples of Hidden Sugars

- Breads
- Pasta
- Crackers
- Biscuits
- Pancakes
- Waffles
- Potato chips
- Mashed potatoes
- Alcohol: wine, beer and hard liquor
- Yogurt (even plain yogurt has 6 to 10 grams per serving size)
- MSG (monosodium glutamate, or modified food starch): check labels and realize that most fast-food restaurants, Peruvian chicken restaurants and Chinese restaurants add MSG, and even non-organic cottage cheese contains it. It raises insulin and acts like sugar.
- Condiments can also have hidden sugars. Find some dressing with less than 1 gram of sugar. Ketchup always has lots of sugar.

Just don't let yourself get excessively hungry between meals. If you feel hungry, you'll be adding healthy fats gradually until you can go longer without having to snack. Also make sure you don't start out eating too much fat if your body is not used to it. Since insulin is the fat switch, we want to keep insulin low by eating less frequent meals, which will heal the insulin dysfunction.

Breakfast

If you are not hungry, don't eat. Some people are hungry later in the morning or even at noon.

But for breakfast you want a combination of protein and fat. You could add some veggies to an omelet, or an avocado, or even some blended veggies. The key is to not consume any refined carbs, juice or sugar—keep these at zero.

I suggest having eggs for breakfast. Get the pasture-raised organic ones if possible. How many? Depending on your size, between 2 and 4. Eggs cooked so the yolk is runny are best but not essential. If you do not like eggs or are allergic to them, you're going to replace them with some other protein: cheese, steak, sardines, fish, chicken, or even a hamburger patty.

Personally, I also add bacon (organic and hormone-free), as it's fatty enough to get me to the next meal with a very low score on the insulin scale. If you don't eat pork, use turkey bacon.

Examples:

- Eggs
- Bacon
- Omelets
- Steak
- High-quality protein shake

I recommend adding a little bit of fat if you have a hard time getting to lunch without a snack: Brie cheese, olives, almond butter, nuts or, my favorite: avocado.

Adding any vegetables to your breakfast is acceptable. These include spinach, tomato, mushrooms, etc. However, no corn or soy.

Lunch

For lunch I normally recommend a salad or veggies eaten first, then some protein. If you add them together, not a problem. Make sure you don't go for lean protein or low-fat *anything*. We want whole-protein food. Eat a moderate amount of protein, from 3 to 6 ounces. Too much will spike insulin; too little will create fatigue. You have to experiment with your body to hit the sweet spot. I do recommend trying to eat your vegetable first because it's easy to overdo it and eat too much protein if you don't have the salad in your stomach. I know some people who can sit down and eat a massive quantity of chicken wings, for example, without becoming full. Eating the salad first seems to satisfy people.

You need to add some healthy fats to be satisfied longer as well. To do this you can include olives, avocado, fatty cheese (like Brie) or almond butter. Your salad or vegetable size needs to be sufficient to satisfy that

4,700 milligram daily requirement for potassium. So a nice 5-cup-size salad would be great. If you can't do that, you can drink your salad.

Examples:
- Salad/vegetable + chicken
- Salad/vegetable + beef
- Salad/vegetable + fish or other seafood

Dinner

For dinner, you can have a meal similar to your lunch, but many people tend to go lower on the protein. If you're doing a big breakfast, you may not be very hungry for dinner. On the other hand, if you skipped breakfast, you might need a big dinner. You can eat your vegetable first, then your protein, then some fat if needed. However, if by morning you're starving, add more fat at night.

You want your dinner to be the last meal of the night. Many people tend to graze at night between dinner and when they go to sleep; not good. It's a mindless habit that needs to be broken by just increasing your awareness. If you want to do a sugar-free dessert AT DINNER, no problem.

Food Intake

You can eat the vegetables listed below in unlimited quantities. Other vegetables not listed are also okay.

Unlimited Vegetables

- alfalfa sprouts
- artichokes
- asparagus
- avocado
- bamboo shoots
- beans
- beets
- bok choy*
- broccoli*
- Brussels sprouts*
- cabbage*
- carrots
- cauliflower*
- celery
- cilantro
- collard greens*
- cucumbers
- dill
- eggplant
- escarole
- garlic
- ginger root
- kale*
- leeks

- lettuce
- mushrooms
- okra
- olives
- onions
- parsley
- peas
- peppers (all)

- pickles (w/out sugar)
- radishes*
- salsa (w/out sugar)
- sauerkraut
- seaweed
- spinach
- squash

- string beans
- sugar snap peas
- Swiss chard
- tomatoes†
- turnip greens*
- turnips*
- water chestnuts
- zucchini

The vegetables in the above chart that are marked with an asterisk are cruciferous and they have a very slight effect of reducing iodine, which is used by the thyroid to make its hormones. This would probably only occur if you ate cruciferous vegetables exclusively, since raw nuts and other foods put back the iodine. But, to be conservative, if you are consuming a moderate to large quantity of cruciferous vegetables every day, add some sea kelp or dulse to your diet—just a small sprinkle on your food or greens. Sea kelp is also supplied in the Cruciferous product recommended in the Resources section. **If you are on thyroid medication, add sea kelp for the iodine.** (See Resources section for more information.)

I recommend a good amount of cruciferous vegetables because of their great ability to improve the liver. The liver is the hub for all fat-burning hormones.

Kale is a superior vegetable. This vegetable is my personal favorite, and I recommend you make a kale shake each day by combining a handful of kale (stems and all), a cup of berries and a glass of water. If your metabolism is slow, instead of berries add liquid stevia (berry flavor). Blend for four minutes and drink up. Kale is one of the best sources of calcium, potassium, manganese and vitamins A and C. It is excellent for the liver and digestive organs. It contains cancer-fighting substances called indoles, which activate detoxifying enzymes in the liver that help neutralize potentially carcinogenic substances. Studies have shown that the plant chemicals in the kale family have a protective effect against the risk of cataracts.‡

---

* Cruciferous: These are a group of vegetables belonging to the cabbage family, named for their tiny cross-shaped flowers.
† Tomatoes are really classified as fruit.
‡ *Source:* George Mateljan Foundation, *The World's Healthiest Foods:* Kale.

One ounce of **broccoli sprouts** contains the same amount of cancer-fighting properties as 1¼ pounds of cooked broccoli.

When a seed starts growing as a sprout, a tremendous amount of nutrition is released from that seed. If your goal is to get healthy and heal the body, sprouts are essential in your diet. Eating small quantities of sprouts is equivalent to eating large quantities of vegetables as far as nutrients are concerned. If you don't like or can't eat a lot of vegetables, then add some daily sprouts to your diet. Put them in your salad each day. You can grow them in a sprouting jar; they are also readily available in health food stores and supermarkets. Don't underestimate these tiny little greens.

The vegetables may be lightly steamed. However, it is recommended that you eat at least 50 percent of them completely raw.

The key is to eat as many of these vegetables as you can, which is hard to do for most people. But you must not bloat or generate gas on this program, and if you do, then switch to other types of vegetables like spring green lettuce, asparagus, string beans, etc.

Dairy

Do not drink milk. You can consume a small amount (3 ounces per day) of organic cottage cheese, Brie cheese, cream cheese, heavy cream, half and half or sour cream within this plan. Butter is okay too, but try to get the grass-fed kind (for example, Kerrygold).

You can also eat grass-fed cheese with meals (no more than 3 ounces per day), or sprinkle some feta cheese on your salad. Kerrygold is an easy-to-find and excellent source of quality grass-fed cheese and butter.

Many people develop mucus from dairy products and/or have allergies. If this happens to you, then avoid dairy products (foods developed from milk). And as a side note, eggs are not considered dairy because they are from chickens.

Don't Eat Starches

Don't eat starchy vegetables, such as french fries, baked potatoes, mashed potatoes, yams and sweet potatoes. Also avoid corn, since most of it is too starchy, has low nutrition and is GMO. This includes avoiding corn chips, tortillas and the million other products containing corn.

Don't Eat Grains

Don't consume breads, pasta, cereal, crackers, biscuits, waffles, muffins, pancakes, rice, rice cakes, donuts, etc., as they readily turn into sugar.

Allergies and Food Sensitivities

Some people are sensitive to sulfur-based vegetables like broccoli. Others are allergic to peanuts. Avoid any foods you are sensitive to. If you are experiencing bloating or gas, you need to consume only vegetables that give you no reaction. If all vegetables seem to cause bloating, you should avoid them for now or eat them cooked.

Salad Dressings

Try to buy dressings that contain no soy oil, no corn oil, and no canola oil. Most of these oils are GMO. The other point is to avoid high-fructose corn syrup, dextrose and cane or beet sugar. Monosodium glutamate (MSG), also known as modified food starch, must be avoided too.

The health food store is your best bet. One recommendation is Bragg salad dressings. As a simple alternative, mix balsamic vinegar and olive oil, or even apple cider vinegar and olive oil, as a dressing.

Tip: Turmeric spice is also recommended for sprinkling on your vegetables. Studies have shown that the combination of this spice with cruciferous vegetables had significant tumor-fighting effects on certain cancers.* I sprinkle it on my salad (kale leaves), or I take cut cauliflower and either steam it or slightly cook it in coconut oil until yellow, then add turmeric on top.

Fruits

Fruits contain way more sugar than vegetables, and for this reason you need to avoid them IF you are trying to lose weight. However, once you achieve your goal weight, I have found that most people can include them back in, in small amounts. In the previous edition of this book I recommended apples and fruits in smaller amounts, but I have changed

---

* *Source:* George Mateljan Foundation, *The World's Healthiest Foods:* Cauliflower.

my recommendations, since even apples contain 19 grams of sugar. I have many clients who, simply by avoiding fruit, finally start losing weight when previously they were stuck.

One of my recommendations is the kale shake, in which you blend kale with one cup of berries. Out of all the fruits, berries contain the least amount of sugar. My opinion of berries is mixed: some people can lose weight with a small quantity of berries and some cannot; so you can test the waters and see if one cup of berries blended in your kale shake will, or will not, be an issue. Try it out and see what happens.

In this book, I talk about eating foods high in nutrients. Certain fruits, especially berries, do contain higher levels of nutrients, so they appear to be on the okay list to eat. The problem can be hidden sugars, which prevent weight loss for someone with a low metabolism; thus we have to consider both of these factors.

The following fruits are off-limits:

- Apples
- Apricots
- Cherries
- Grapefruit
- Grapes
- Kiwis
- Melons
- Nectarines
- Oranges
- Peaches
- Pears
- Persimmons
- Pineapples
- Plums

These fruits are okay:

- Lemons
- Limes
- Berries (try them to see if they influence your weight or not)
- Tomatoes (in small amounts)

Animal Proteins

Depending on your size, consume 3 to 6 ounces of animal protein (eggs, fish, meat, chicken, etc.) with meals. This recommendation is different from my statements in the previous edition of this book.

There is one point I want to bring up regarding eliminating animal protein and animal fat from the diet completely, which can create some problems. I have the advantage of observing many clients and their reactions to all sorts of diets. For example: A few clients, after implementing dietary changes recommended in the documentary *Forks over Knives*, which promotes pure vegetarianism (no animal proteins or animal fats), lost several teeth. Another lost his hair.

These problems were due to cutting out all animal protein and fat. Animal protein is a complete protein. Most of the human body is made out of protein, and animal fats give us fat-soluble vitamins (A, D, E, K). The connective tissue that holds your teeth in place and the hair on your head is made from protein. Cutting these foods out completely can starve your body of the raw materials needed to build body proteins. I am not completely against a vegetarian diet for some people. However, you have to know what you are doing and you need to know where to get ALL your basic nutrients, including fat-soluble vitamins and the complete amino-acid profile. I frequently ask vegans, "Where do you get your fat-soluble vitamins, like vitamin A?" They respond that they get them from vegetables. Actually there is no active form of vitamin A in vegetables, only pre-vitamin A, which converts to around just 4 percent of the active form.

I am aware of the philosophical arguments against eating animals and the debate on what we were designed to eat. But if we work backwards and first look at what nutrient requirements we have and then what foods fit those requirements, we can come up with the best diet. The purpose of food is to get nutrients, right? So my general recommendation is to include at least some animal protein, such as fish, eggs, etc. If eating animal proteins is against your religion or against your philosophy, then do some research first before you jump in. Many so-called vegetarians are really grainarians or fruitarians; they gain lots of weight eating whole grains and drinking carrot juice, which contains an overload of hidden sugars. And some do not consume enough actual vegetables.

On this program you are consuming plenty of greens, with some animal protein and fat. Adding fat is a necessity for required nutrients and to be satisfied without triggering fat-making hormones like insulin. For those people who have either a missing gallbladder or a sluggish gallbladder, no matter how much fat they eat, they are still hungry. In such cases, add Gallbladder Formula to your meal to better absorb the fat you're already eating. The most important action is to avoid feeling too unsatisfied, since this leads to continual snacking.

The animal proteins that I recommend are covered in the following sections.

Fish (wild-caught) and Seafood

Seafood (oysters, shrimp, mussels, squid, scallops, lobster or crab)
Healthiest fish:
Tuna (trawl- or pole-caught), salmon, sardines, trout, halibut (Pacific), perch, cod, tilapia, flounder and sashimi/sushi (without rice)
Avoid bluefin tuna, orange roughy, farm-raised salmon, mahi-mahi and Atlantic halibut.

Grass-Fed, Organic Meats

Beef, lamb, pork (pasture-raised, organic), buffalo, and chicken and turkey in limited amounts due to processing—more information follows. Organ meats like liver are good (must be organic).

Pork, chicken or turkey should never be consumed in the overly processed form, with added preservatives like nitrates. If you consume bacon, sausage or ham, ensure that it's nitrate-free, organic, and even grass-fed if you can find it. Better yet, try to get it sugar-free. Pork is good for people who are diabetic or insulin resistant (prediabetic) because of the higher fat, which allows them to go longer without eating. I buy my pork at the farmers' market and the health food store, NOT at a convenience store.

Many chickens and turkeys are fed GMO feed that contains formaldehyde. So, at the very minimum, consume non-GMO poultry, but preferably get organic and pasture-raised.

Eggs

Buy chicken eggs that are pasture-raised and organic. Duck eggs are even better.

I recommend eggs for breakfast, but make sure you consume the yolk and all. The yolk contains lecithin, the antidote to cholesterol.

Do not overeat animal proteins—eat just the right amount to satisfy your hunger, which means around 3 to 6 ounces. Overeating will stress the liver and convert protein to fat. Fish is an excellent source of protein on this program, and raw proteins are more easily digested, causing less liver stress than cooked proteins.

Vegetarian Proteins

It is more difficult to find vegetarian proteins for our purpose because vegetables tend to come with carbohydrates. However, the proteins below are helpful:

- Spirulina
- Protein powder (pea, hemp, brown rice)
- Organic fermented soy (smaller amounts): tofu, tempeh
- Seeds (sunflower, sesame, pumpkin)
- Sprouted beans
- Lentils
- Mushrooms
- Almond butter
- Nuts
- Nutritional yeast
- Hummus

Fats

This is the big variable. People always ask, "How many grams or ounces of fat can I eat?" That's a hard one, since you have many variables: bile reserve, digestive strength, age, history of eating fats, liver function and so on. You will have to test the waters, but between 20 and 40 grams is about average. Start out with a small piece of Brie cheese (2 to 3 ounces) or a small handful of nuts or maybe a teaspoon of peanut butter after each meal. But always eat your fats with the meal, not as a snack.

Below are some examples of fats you can choose.

Fat	Amount	Grams of Fat
Nuts (pecans, almonds, pistachios, walnuts)	1 oz (10 nuts)	20 grams
Butter (from grass-fed cows; Kerrygold is good)	1 Tbsp	11 grams
Seeds (sunflower, pumpkin or sesame)	1 oz	14 grams
Peanut butter or almond butter (no added sugars)	1 Tbsp	10 grams
Bacon (no nitrates or hormones)	1 slice	3 grams
Coconut butter or oil	1 Tbsp	14 grams
Sour cream, cream cheese, whole cream (organic)	1 Tbsp	5 grams
Olive oil or olives	1 Tbsp	14 grams
Avocado	1 whole	30 grams
Cheese (try to eat Brie or other fattier cheese)	3 oz	28 grams
Grass-fed hot dogs	1 link	10 grams

Avoid these fats: trans fats, margarine, soy oil, corn oil and canola oil.

Also, realize most proteins in their whole form have fat, so you'll have to take that into consideration.

Raw Nuts and Seeds

Eat nuts and seeds only with meals. Raw pecans, almonds and walnuts are great choices; however, sunflower seeds and pumpkin seeds are even better. Some people could be allergic to nuts or will experience bloating if the nuts and seeds are not germinated (soaked overnight in water), and in this section I will explain how to do this.

Acceptable nuts and seeds:

- Almonds

- Walnuts
- Hazelnuts
- Pecans
- Pine nuts
- Pistachios
- Peanuts
- Brazil nuts
- Sunflower seeds
- Pumpkin seeds
- Unsweetened peanut butter
- Tahini butter

Pecans

- Rich in manganese, magnesium, phosphorus, zinc, vitamin B_1 and vitamin E
- Extremely low on the insulin index (5 percent)
- Nutrient-dense healthy fats to help satiety (feeling full)
- Can decrease bad cholesterol (LDL) and increase good cholesterol (HDL)
- Can help patients with insulin resistance

Stale or old nuts that have been sitting around for months must not be eaten. Keeping nuts in a sealed container or bag and in the refrigerator is a smart idea.

IMPORTANT NOTE: Many people, when starting a new eating plan, eat way too many nuts. It's easy to overeat them, especially pistachios. This will create stress on the gallbladder, which then causes right-shoulder pain, right-scapula tightness or right-neck tightness. This is due to irritation of the phrenic nerve (connecting the gallbladder area up to the right shoulder and neck), which is influenced by a congested or sluggish gallbladder. If the nerve is irritated, it can even cause misalignment of the lower neck and pinch nerves that go down to the right arm and hand, or even into the right jaw. I have had so many people come in with right-wrist, hand, finger or even elbow pain who have no idea that the root cause is the gallbladder. Do not overeat nuts. Start with ¼ cup per day.

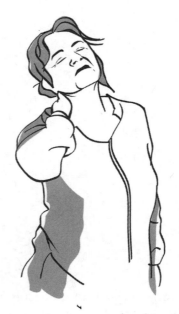

Roasted nuts, like peanuts, create the biggest problem in larger quantities, and raw peanuts just don't taste good. You could have fewer peanuts and small amounts of peanut butter, providing you eat raw nuts as well and make sure the peanut butter doesn't contain added sugar or hydrogenated oils. I like dipping celery in a mixture of 50 percent peanut butter and 50 percent tahini (sesame seed) butter.

Nuts and seeds grow into trees and plants. Enzymes within them activate this growth (enzymes are substances that cause and increase the speed of chemical reactions). However, inherently, nuts and seeds also have what are called *enzyme inhibitors*, which are tiny locks that prevent growth. *Inhibit* means "to hold back or keep from some action," and enzyme inhibitors keep enzyme activity from happening until the right condition exists for the nut or seed to grow into a tree or plant capable of reproduction. The main element that establishes this right condition for growth is water.

Sometimes consuming nuts and seeds in sufficient quantity can cause unpleasant heaviness in the abdomen, even bloating and gas. This is because of the enzyme inhibitors. In other words, eating nuts and seeds without first inactivating their enzyme inhibitors forces the pancreas to work overtime, releasing lots of its *own* enzymes. A stressed pancreas will slow digestion and cause bloating. When this happens over an extended period of time, you start to lose your enzyme reserves, and without all of your enzymes, you'll have a hard time digesting foods like cruciferous vegetables. People mistake this condition for an allergy to the cruciferous vegetables. Studies performed on animals that were fed nuts with enzyme inhibitors intact showed a doubling in size of the animals' pancreases, stunted growth, impaired health and decreased enzyme reserves.

So, how do we handle this problem?

Squirrels bury their nuts in the ground to activate the enzymes and deactivate the enzyme inhibitors. (That's one thing you could do, but first let me get my camera!) You could also cook the nuts and seeds, although the heat would destroy the nutritional value, since enzymes are very sensitive to any heat. This is why you should try to consume at least 50 percent of your nuts and seeds raw. The other half can be roasted, but just make sure there are no added sweeteners or MSG (or modified corn starch). The best thing to do is activate the enzymes in the nuts and seeds to start the process of germination (*germinate* means "to cause to sprout or grow"). Here is the way you do this:

1. Soak your seeds and nuts in filtered or spring water overnight—12 hours is ideal—in a covered glass or metal container. Cheesecloth makes a good cover.

2. In the morning, rinse the seeds and nuts several times to drain off the fluid containing the enzyme inhibitors.

3. Let them dry on some surface like a wire strainer that will allow air to permeate. They will stay moist, but you can dry them out either in the oven or in a dehydrator. If you use an oven, set the heat as low as possible (170 degrees F) until the nuts or seeds are free of moisture. A dehydrator set at 95 to 100 degrees F will take 12 to 24 hours, and at this lower temperature the enzymes will stay intact.

4. Start eating. You are now consuming live superfood. This process of germination will not only take stress off your digestive system, it will also increase the availability of additional active enzymes, vitamins and minerals, such as calcium, magnesium, iron, copper and zinc.

5. Store what you don't eat in a glass container in your refrigerator to increase shelf life and freshness, as germinated seeds and nuts do not keep as long.

Beans/Lentils/Legumes

Unfortunately beans, lentils and legumes tend to have a few more carbs than we want; however, I do still recommend them for vegetarians, as they contain some protein. The bean that has the most protein is the soybean; but given that 90 percent of all soy in the U.S. is GMO, you should avoid soy unless you consume non-GMO (or organic). Soy is also very estrogenic. I am not against having a small number of fermented, non-GMO, organic soy products in your diet (tofu, tempeh and miso); but never consume soy protein isolate, the main protein in a lot of the prepackaged food camouflaged as weight-loss products. There are too many side effects, and we were never meant to digest soy protein isolate.

I have no problem with your eating beans, hummus and lentils in small amounts—as in ½ to 1 cup per day. I do not believe that they will cause weight gain; however, they can slow your ability to lose weight. Hummus is good to use as your dip for cut vegetables (celery, tomatoes, red and green peppers, etc.).

Supplement Intake

There is one type of supplement recommended for those people who just can't seem to get enough variety of vegetables: a special greens product. This nutrient will supply the raw material for the liver to rejuvenate as well as build up your cells' potassium reserves.

It is difficult to find supplements containing most of the cruciferous greens, so I personally created a high-quality organic cruciferous food concentrate with several additional vegetables for other health benefits. It's called **Organic Cruciferous Superfood**. It contains an organic blend of cruciferous and other nutrient-dense vegetables, including organic asparagus, beets, Brussels sprouts, cabbage, cauliflower, collard greens, kale, parsley, radish, garlic, sea kelp and turmeric. I have removed broccoli, since it tended to bloat people more than any other vegetable. All these vegetables are extremely beneficial for the liver.

The other advantage of this supplement is that it contains organic sea kelp, which has iodine and will counter any iodine-depleting effects the cruciferous vegetables have.

Apple Cider Vinegar & Lemon Drink

You will be drinking a mixture containing apple cider vinegar and some lemon (either an actual squeezed lemon or premade lemon juice). You may want to add a few drops of stevia if you don't like the sourness.

To prepare this drink, mix together the following ingredients:

- 1 tablespoon of apple cider vinegar
- 1 tablespoon of lemon juice or 1 whole lemon (my favorite bottled lemon juice is Italian Volcano Organic Lemon Juice, if you can find it)
- 1 glass of spring or filtered water (8 to 10 ounces)

Drink it with a straw to protect your teeth!

Starting out, it would be good to take this drink three times per day with meals. Some people either love it or hate it. If you hate it, avoid it—your body is telling you that you don't need it.

Apple cider vinegar can help you improve insulin function, especially insulin resistance.

Lemons prevent the development of kidney stones and promote normal immune function because they are high in natural vitamin C. Lemon juice also helps contract the liver (astringent). And lemon is necessary to help counter the potential negative effects from oxylates in the kale and spinach you may be eating, which could cause kidney stones.

Most people's bodies are not acid enough, and this goes against what "they say." There's a big push to "alkalize" people. This confusion has stemmed from not understanding body pH.

Each part of the body has a different pH (acid/alkaline level).

Stomach: 1.5 (extremely acidic)
Saliva: 6.4 (slightly acidic)
Blood: 7.4 (slightly alkaline)
Pancreatic juice: 8.0 (alkaline)
Urine: 5.8 (acidic)
Small intestine: 8.0 (alkaline)
Large intestine: 5.0 (acidic)

So when someone says we are all too acid, what part are they talking about? Usually they are basing the pH on urine, which is supposed to be acidic anyway.

But if a person has more of an Adrenal body type due to stress, they will generally be on the overly alkaline side; and I am talking about the blood pH. Why? Because high cortisol causes a loss of acids through the urine and leaves you with alkalosis (overly alkaline). This is a general statement; but rather than do expensive testing to find your exact pH, it would be much easier to take some apple cider vinegar in your water and see if you feel better.

Symptoms of pH Imbalance

Too Acid

- Chest pain
- Palpitations
- Headaches
- Anxiety
- Muscle weakness
- Bone pain
- Joint pain
- Air hunger

Too Alkaline

- Muscle twitches (tetany)
- Allergies
- Muscle spasms
- Muscle cramps
- Muscle weakness
- Dehydration
- Muscle pain
- Difficulty breathing

A Few Guidelines

1. Refrain from eating anything that is not in this chapter. So many foods have hidden sugars, and one of my goals is to raise awareness of these: protein bars, vanilla yogurt or plain yogurt, juice, sports drinks, and the list goes on and on.

2. Avoid tap water. Spring and filtered water are best. Personally, I do drink a lot of mineral water (San Pellegrino and Gerolsteiner Mineral Water, both of which are carbonated mineral waters).

3. Naturally caffeine-free herbal teas are totally acceptable.

4. If you can avoid coffee, that would be great. However, many people need to do this gradually to avoid having a headache for two weeks. Try to only drink one small cup in the morning and drink organic

coffee if possible. If you use cream, use organic, or better yet, grass-fed. If you normally add sugar, use xylitol instead.

5. I would also avoid alcohol for now. A drink (including wine, beer and hard liquor) can set your liver back for a few days. As a substitute, I recommend kombucha tea. It has a similar texture to beer and wine and is carbonated. Pour it in a wine glass and pretend it's alcohol—it should give you a calming effect.

6. If you are currently exercising, you can continue—but not if you aren't sleeping and have fatigue. You'll find a lot more information on this when you get to the chapter on exercise, chapter 17. The worse the sleep, the more you should do low-intensity exercise: walking, yoga, etc.

7. If possible, try not to go to restaurants too much, as the result is too unpredictable. Socializing with friends can easily tempt you to consume alcohol, bread and dessert.

Three-Day Sample of What to Eat

Monday

Breakfast	**Lunch**	**Dinner**
Apple cider vinegar and lemon drink	*Apple cider vinegar and lemon drink*	*Apple cider vinegar and lemon drink*
• 2 to 3 eggs and bacon	• Large salad (5 cups)	• Vegetables: asparagus and mushrooms (4 cups)
	• Steak (3 to 6 ounces)	• Fish (3 to 6 ounces)
	• ½ avocado	• Pecans (handful)

Tuesday

Breakfast	**Lunch**	**Dinner**
Apple cider vinegar and lemon drink	*Apple cider vinegar and lemon drink*	*Apple cider vinegar and lemon drink*
• 2-egg omelet: spinach (1 cup) with cheese (3 ounces)	• Spinach salad (7 cups)	• Steamed cabbage (2 cups)
	• Tuna (3 to 6 ounces)	• Beef burger patty (3 to 6 ounces)
	• Olives (½ cup)	• 3 tsp peanut butter

Wednesday

Breakfast

Apple cider vinegar and lemon drink

- 2 to 3 eggs with sausage
- ½ avocado

Lunch

Apple cider vinegar and lemon drink

- Kale shake (5 cups kale blended with 1 cup berries)
- Chicken (3 to 6 ounces)
- Brie cheese (3 ounces)

Dinner

Apple cider vinegar and lemon drink

- Steamed veggies (5 cups)
- Shrimp (3 to 6 ounces)
- ¼ cup pistachios

NO SNACKING—adjust the fat you take with meals to allow you to go longer without being hungry!

Quick Healthy Small Meals

- Button mushrooms sautéed in butter
- Celery with almond butter
- Cut vegetables dipped in guacamole (avocado, onion, tomato, cumin, mayonnaise, lemon juice and garlic)
- Pickles and olives (for people who crave salt)
- Cooked cabbage with garlic and onion
- Cut tomato with cheese (3 ounces)
- Cucumber slices in dill dip
- Celery with hummus
- Celery dipped in a mixture of peanut butter and tahini butter (sesame seeds)
- Spaghetti squash with tomato sauce (low-sugar)
- Cheese melted over broccoli
- Fried eggplant (in olive oil)
- Slightly cooked cauliflower with turmeric spice
- Tomato and basil leaf with cheese (3 ounces)

Salad Ideas

- Tomato, avocado, black pepper, basil leaves, sprouts
- Cabbage (shredded), almonds, kale
- Steamed or pickled beets, cucumbers, onion (sautéed)
- Lettuce, lemon juice, kidney beans, sprouts
- Chickpeas, romaine lettuce, black olives
- Bok choy, asparagus, sugar snap peas, carrots, sunflower seeds
- Cabbage, celery, parsley, cashews, sprouts
- Steamed spinach, peas, ginger root, lentils, lime juice
- Pinto beans, tomatoes, avocado, olives, red cabbage
- Cabbage, sautéed mushrooms, cauliflower sautéed in butter or coconut oil until slightly brown
- Cauliflower sautéed in butter or coconut oil until slightly brown, spinach, carrots, broccoli
- Cauliflower sautéed in butter or coconut oil until slightly brown, hummus
- Black-eyed peas, kidney beans, bell pepper, onion, parsley
- Red cabbage, cut pears, shredded carrots,
- Green pepper, cucumbers, carrots, kale, sprouts
- Broccoli with ranch dip, artichoke hearts
- Black olives, celery, lemon juice, mayonnaise
- Baby spinach, sprouts, celery, beets (raw, not canned)
- Kale, papaya, avocado, black olives

Concentrated Nutrition

There are receptors in your digestive system that signal the brain and tell it when to feel hungry and when to be satisfied. When you consume highly concentrated nutrients, the body's hunger centers are easily satisfied, resulting in fewer cravings and less hunger. This is why you can eat a lot of refined "empty nutrition" bread or other carbohydrate, since carbohydrates do not trigger the brain hunger centers as readily. The reason your cravings will go away on this program is because the body is getting all the nutrition it needs. Cravings only occur when you are missing some nutrients.

What to Expect

As you implement this program, you should notice your cravings decreasing. This means insulin is healing and you are less insulin resistant. With a bit more time, you should have zero cravings and you'll feel less hungry. This is because you will be burning fat and less sugar fuel. You have to realize that it takes a good two weeks, at least, for your body to adapt to fat burning and make new cellular structures and enzymes. It could take six weeks for some people. Your body goes through a transformation so it can run on a different fuel—this is amazing.

The new machine (your fat-burning machine) needs certain nutrients to do its job. Without these nutrients a person can become a bit more tired. If this happens, add some extra B vitamins from nutritional yeast, preferably non-fortified (obtainable from your health food store or Amazon.com). You are not detoxing; you are just missing vitamins. The energy factories in your cells require lots of B vitamins.

You will most definitely lose water weight at first—in fact, anything over two pounds per week is fluid loss. If this happens, ensure that your vegetable consumption stays high so as to maintain your electrolytes (minerals). Also realize that it takes time to get healthy. Even if you lose nothing, understand that the first step is "get healthy," right? In fact, I always tell people to focus on restoring their sleep, energy, stress tolerance and digestion, and reducing cravings. The weight loss always follows.

There also might be weeks when you lose weight and then weeks when you stop losing weight. If this happens when your eating habits stay the same, the cause could be stress, your sleep quality, or some other change. If nothing has changed, chances are you are gaining more muscle, which weighs more than fat. Your best indicator for actual fat loss is your clothing size, especially around your midsection. Are your clothes fitting better? Is your stomach shrinking? If so, it's working.

What's the Next Step after Two Weeks?

At the end of 14 days, you want to start enhancing your program for your primary body type. Each body type needs specific things to keep weight loss going and to accelerate progress.

Based on your results from the quiz in chapter 4, please go to the section for *your* body type in the next chapter and use it to tweak your eating plan.

12

Tailor-Making Your Eating to Your Body Type

My last edition was too complex regarding what to eat for your body type. This version is much simpler. Start with the basic eating plan, and then after two weeks tweak it until you notice seven health factors improving, which I will explain below.

All four body types need the same key basic healing foods. However, adjustments will be needed based on your primary body type. This means adjustments to proteins, fats, nutrients and the type of carbohydrates you eat as well as a few other things.

Your weight is merely one indicator of health, and actually low on the list; it's the last improvement people see. Yet most people expect it to be the first thing to improve—whoops!

Your goal should go beyond just weight loss and include enhancing the following seven health factors:

1. Energy
2. Sleep
3. Stress tolerance
4. Reduced cravings
5. Digestion
6. Reduced inflammation
7. Reduced waist size

It's time to enhance the results you are getting. Once you have determined your specific body type, there are various additions or changes you can make to your basic eating plan to increase your results. I have listed them in the following sections. Many people are a combination of several body types; so the thing to do is find the type that contains more of your symptoms than the others and start there. If you get great improvements, then stick with that. If not, make changes based on another body type. If you are still stuck, you can always call my office and chat with one of my trained health coaches.

Adrenal

There are a few tweaks if you have an Adrenal body type. There are food tweaks, and specific stress-reducing body techniques that I recommend as well.

Dietary Proteins

An overactive adrenal creates excess cortisol. This is the hormone that breaks down protein (for example, muscles) in your body. Adrenal body types need more protein than all other body types; this means increasing your dietary protein, but don't get too crazy. Instead of 3 ounces of protein per meal, you may need 6 or 7 ounces of protein per meal.

Dietary Fats

The other variable with the Adrenal body type is adjusting your fats. Your adrenal hormones are made out of fat, and a low-fat diet will not help the adrenals. Again, we're not going to go crazy dumping massive amounts of fat into your system, but generally you need a good amount of fat in the diet. Always gradually increase your fats because the digestive system, and especially your gallbladder, needs to adapt to the increased demand. Make sure you consume the fats with a meal and not between meals.

Nutrients

The most important nutrients for the adrenals are potassium, B vitamins and vitamin C.

With overactive adrenals, you will lose potassium. Since this mineral is a physiological relaxer, people may become edgy and irritated without enough potassium. Your body requires huge quantities of this mineral, not to mention the extra needs due to your adrenals dumping excess potassium through the kidneys. You must ensure that your intake is at least equal to your output. For potassium, consume 7 to 10 cups of veggies or salad.

B vitamins are in many foods, but adding a teaspoon of nutritional yeast each day will help ensure that you get enough. Just make sure it's nutritional yeast though, not brewer's yeast. Sugar and refined grains (breads, pasta, cereals, etc.) all deplete your B vitamins. Stress depletes B vitamins. In my Stress & Cortisol Relief I have included a complete whole-food B-vitamin/adrenal-support complex; it's great at releasing that internal feeling of nervous stress and tension, which can come from a B-vitamin deficiency.

Your adrenals store a lot of vitamin C and use it as a precursor (raw material) for making adrenal hormones. Most vitamin C sold is made synthetically as ascorbic acid. This is just the antioxidant part. I would only recommend taking synthetic vitamin C if you were using it for a short-term detox, but not as a maintenance product.

If you're getting 7 to 10 cups of vegetables or salad per day, you will also get all your vitamin C requirements—and kill two birds with one stone. Vegetables give you the complete vitamin C complex.

pH and Your Adrenals

One of the problems with the Adrenal type is pH. Adrenal body types tend to turn more alkaline over time. If you want to know why and have some background in chemistry, it is because an overactive adrenal causes a loss of the hydrogen ion (H+). And H+ is an acid. When you lose acids, you become alkaline. So, taking apple cider vinegar in liquid or pills is a good thing to help balance the pH back to its normal range.

Stress-Reducing Techniques

The acupressure techniques in chapter 16 are meant for the Adrenal body type. Releasing body stress will greatly help your adrenals, and no weight-loss program that I know of addresses the body-stress factor. Using my stress-releasing techniques is like getting rid of the open applications on your desktop computer. Your stress accumulates over time and the body holds on to it, thus slowing your ability to lose weight. People who have had minimal stress in their lives rarely have a problem losing weight.

Exercise

Adrenal body types need low-intensity exercise; nothing to overstress the body. Walking is great, yoga is good, and even Pilates will work. The key is to adjust exercise based on your ability to recover. More on this in the exercise chapter—chapter 17.

Liver

Dietary Proteins

The more damaged the liver, the less protein it can process (deal with). Typically the Liver body type needs the smallest quantities of protein. I am going to recommend 3 ounces per meal. Some Liver types do much better on vegetarian proteins, which you may want to try but it's not a requirement. This could include pea protein, spirulina and sprouted lentils.

High-protein diets are not good for the Liver body type.

Dietary Fats

The liver and gallbladder use bile to digest fat. Adding too much fat can overwhelm the liver and gallbladder and create lots of bloating, belching and burping. For this reason, go light with fats, but don't completely eliminate them. Whereas the Adrenal type needs a lot more, Liver body types can only tolerate about half the fats recommended for the Adrenal type. Yet it actually takes saturated fats to cause the liver and gallbladder to release bile; so going completely fat-free can shrivel up your gallbladder and bile supply.

There are certain fats that are more tolerated than others. Medium-chain fats like coconut oil and butter are perfect; whereas vegetable oils like corn and soy are more of a strain on the liver and gallbladder.

Carbohydrates

Refined carbs and sugars are really stressful on the liver. The absolute best carbohydrate for the liver is vegetables. You will not be able to fix or repair the liver without consuming large amounts of vegetables; sorry to break this to you. Vegetables have fiber for your microbes to consume; they have vitamins and minerals and an additional factor called phytonutrients. These are plant-based health-benefiting nutrients that go beyond just vitamins and minerals. For example, one is called sulforaphane. This natural compound helps to turn poisons in the liver to harmless particles—amazing. It contains reparative factors and preventative factors, especially against cancer. Vegetables have hundreds and hundreds of naturally occurring phytonutrients.

At the top of the list, the cruciferous type of vegetable ranks number one in contributions to liver health. Cruciferous vegetables include kale, cauliflower, cabbage, broccoli, bok choy, arugula, Brussels sprouts, collard greens and mustard greens.

Nutrients

The most important minerals for the liver are sulfur and selenium. Also important are certain B vitamins: B_2, B_3 and B_6. You can get all these in cruciferous vegetables. Another great nutrient to strip fat off the liver is choline. This can easily be found at any health food store or online.

Liver Technique

The following acupressure technique for the liver and gallbladder will help improve circulation and blood flow and reduce organ congestion. Rarely does anyone ever massage these areas. Why not? People get body work on their muscles; why not work on the organs too? The only caution is to start out gently and massage within your tolerance. Sometimes these areas can be tense and tender, but normally they should be relaxed and not tender. And one more point: If you have had your gallbladder removed, I recommend massaging ONLY the opposite side, the area around the pancreas.

Below is a diagram showing how to do it.

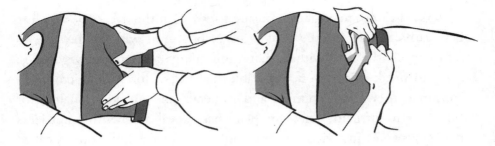

Also do the opposite side and massage the pancreas area.

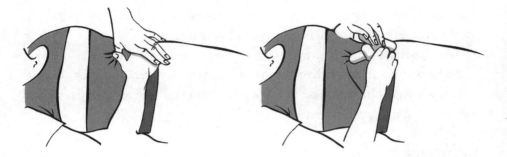

Ovary

Dietary Proteins

The required protein amount is moderate for the Ovary body type; however, since the Ovary type only applies to women, generally speaking dietary proteins are needed in lesser amounts than for men. Typically 3 to 4 ounces of protein works fine. But the more important factor about protein is the need for quality. This means "without hormones."

The main hormone that is used to increase milk production in cows is a hormone called rBST. It will increase milk output by 10 percent and was originally created by the company Monsanto. rBST is a GMO product. It is banned by the European Union. It triggers other hormones that are linked to increasing your risk of getting cancer, especially breast cancer.

Organic means grown without chemical fertilizers, pesticides and sprays. These chemicals can influence the female glands and hormones.

Grass-fed animal products are best, since grass-fed cows and other farm animals provide the most nutrition and are GMO-free. If the label does not say "Grass-fed," then it means they were grain-fed (corn and soy), and typically with GMO grain unless it says "Organic." The best choice is grass-fed and organic, which is more expensive but ideal. If you can't swing it, at the very least get products that are hormone-free (without rBST).

Wild-caught means that fish and seafood are caught in the ocean. Many farm-raised fish are given hormones too; so avoid farm-raised fish and get wild-caught.

Dairy (including milk, yogurt, kefir, cream, sour cream, half and half, cheese, etc.) should minimally be free of hormones (no rBST). You can see this on labels as "Milk from cows not treated with rBST."

If you buy organic foods, you can know at least that there are regulations banning GMOs. Again, the problem with GMOs is the heavy quantity of the pesticide glyphosate that is used in the grains (soy and corn) the animals consume.

Pasture-raised is another important term; it means the animal is allowed to go out in the grass. This is very different from *free-range* or *cage-free*, which doesn't guarantee the animals get to experience grass.

Personally, I buy organic pasture-raised eggs, which are the best, and I try to get them at the farmers' market.

Dietary Fats

The amount of dietary fats an Ovary body type can eat is moderate—higher than the Thyroid and Liver types but a bit less than the Adrenal type. If you are eating butter, make sure it's grass-fed butter (example: Kerrygold).

Nutrients

A vitally important nutrient for the ovaries and other female glands is iodine. Like the Thyroid body type, the Ovary body type needs iodine. In fact, iodine acts as an estrogen regulator; it helps lower excess estrogen. Iodine can shrink an estrogen-created cyst on the ovary, uterus or breast (as in fibrocystic breasts). I prefer to get iodine from sea kelp. A little sea kelp goes a long way.

Other nutrients needed by the Ovary type are certain phytonutrients, which are present in cruciferous vegetables. These nutrients are anti-estrogenic; they protect you against the harmful effects of estrogen. Cruciferous vegetables do deplete iodine. To prevent this, I recommend adding sea kelp to your diet if you eat cruciferous vegetables. My Cruciferous Superfood product has a blend of cruciferous vegetables and sea kelp to help you ensure that no iodine deficiency occurs. The Estrogen Balance formula is also used for excess estrogen and contains a concentrated ingredient from cruciferous vegetables. (See the Resources section for both of these.)

Thyroid

The interesting thing about the Thyroid body type is that thyroid difficulty is usually a secondary problem. Most thyroid conditions are really the result of either a liver/gallbladder issue or an overly active ovary issue, or even an adrenal problem. This is why so many people see no change when they are diagnosed with hypothyroidism and they are put on thyroid hormones.

The thyroid hormones get activated (start working) as they pass through the liver and gallbladder. If there is a problem with the liver or gallbladder, then the thyroid hormone T4 does not turn into T3, and regardless of how much hormone you have, it just doesn't work. Having a lot of inactive thyroid hormone will keep you fat, tired and constipated.

People with gallbladder or liver problems (constipation, bloating, right-shoulder pain) or who have had their gallbladders removed tend to have thyroid deficiencies.

Excessive estrogen can block the thyroid. This is why many women develop hypothyroidism after becoming pregnant. Pregnancy dramatically spikes estrogen.

In the case of the low (hypo)–thyroid autoimmune condition called Hashimoto's, or even the high (hyper)–thyroid case known as Graves' (another autoimmune condition), the adrenals are usually behind the problem. Every autoimmune condition I have ever seen occurred after some stress event or severe loss. Excess stress equals an overactive adrenal.

How can we know which real cause it is?

Ask yourself, "When did I develop a thyroid problem, and what occurred just before?" Was it due to an estrogen spike? Or something wrong with the gallbladder, like having the gallbladder removed? Or did it occur after a stress event, like divorce or loss of a loved one, or even some physical trauma?

It would be best to focus on fixing the real cause of the thyroid problem; however, you should also support your thyroid at the same time.

If the thyroid problem is due to
- Liver or gallbladder: Take the Gallbladder Formula.
- High estrogen: Take the Organic Cruciferous Superfood.
- Autoimmune (adrenal related): Take the Adrenal support.

See Resources section for more info.

Dietary Proteins

The amount of protein the Thyroid body type can handle is low. This is due to the metabolism being slow; too much protein will overload the digestion.

A very good source of protein for a Thyroid type is seafood and ocean fish. Why? Because of the added iodine and the ease with which these proteins are digested.

Dietary Fats

The amount of fat a Thyroid type should have needs to be lower too. A Thyroid type has a slow metabolism and doesn't have the capacity to digest a lot of fat. Coconut oil is a great fat for Thyroid types.

Nutrients

The most important two minerals for the thyroid would be iodine and selenium. Iodine is what the thyroid hormones are made from and selenium helps in the conversion. Sea kelp is the best source for these. Take 1 to 2 capsules in the early morning—but never before bed, as it could give you too much energy. The reason I like taking sea kelp for the thyroid instead of straight iodine is that it contains a blend of all the minerals and trace minerals.

Thyroid Technique

There is an acupressure technique recommended for the thyroid that involves pressure points on the opposite side of the thyroid, in the back part of your neck. It tends to increase circulation into the front of your neck and thyroid. See page 238 for more information.

As you attempt to tweak your eating further with the above recommendations, you will also want to use various symptoms to know if your health is getting better; they will act as guides, telling you what to do.

How to Know If Things Are Working

There are various symptoms that you can use to know what's going on inside your body.

Insulin Resistance Improvement

If you notice that any of these are improving, your insulin is healing:

1. Feeling satisfied after eating
2. No more cravings for sweets
3. Can go a long time without eating—or being hungry
4. Energy after eating

One small point about being tired after meals: this could also mean your stomach is not acid enough, resulting in undigested proteins. Add apple cider vinegar with water to correct this, or take the Digest Formula before you eat (see Resources section).

Hypoglycemia (low blood sugars) and Dietary Protein

There is another condition related to blood sugars called hypoglycemia (low blood sugars). This is also a prediabetic condition. It is usually created by eating too much refined sugar and carbs. Protein is the food that will correct this condition. Dietary protein triggers hormones (glucagon and growth hormone) that release stored sugars (glycogen), raising the sugar level to normal.

You will use the following symptoms to know that you are consuming the right amount of protein:

1. No longer irritable between meals
2. Body doesn't feel cold
3. Better and more stable mood
4. Less tired and more energy after eating

Adjust your proteins to improve these symptoms. If you have too much protein, you can also get tired, bloated or constipated and sleep less well.

Basic Rules of Eating for Hormone Health

Avoid sugar, fruits, grains and starches

Avoid sweeteners, candy, juice and actual sugar—and this also includes honey, agave, brown sugar, raw sugar, malt sugar, date sugar and every other type of sugar. The only acceptable sugars are xylitol, erythritol, stevia and glycerol (from coconuts).

Avoid fruits—all fruits except lemons and limes. The fruit that has the highest amount of sugar is the apple. Yes, I used to recommend apples until I found out they have 19 grams of sugar—way too high. Berries in small amounts may be okay unless your metabolism is super low. Also avoid dried fruit, as in raisins, figs and dates; and especially avoid canned fruit. Fruits tend to stop weight loss but don't so much cause you to gain weight. So once you hit your goal, you can add fruits back into your diet.

Avoid grains—breads, pasta, crackers, cereal and others. This also includes oatmeal and rice. Once you hit your goal, you can have wild rice.

Avoid starches—potatoes, yams and corn. Also avoid sweet potatoes. Potatoes are a great way to gain weight without creating nutritional deficiencies, as you would if you ate cakes and cookies. When you achieve your goal weight, you can add them back in.

Avoid beans and lentils—except hummus. Beans and lentils can slow weight loss due to their high content of carbohydrates. Once you achieve your weight-loss goal, you can add them back in. EXCEPTION: If you are a vegetarian, go ahead and consume beans and lentils.

Avoid alcohol—beer, wine, hard liquor and Champagne.

Consume lots of nutrient-dense vegetables

This includes all the non-starchy vegetables, salads, leafy greens and cruciferous. Eat them in their whole form, mainly raw and some steamed. Brussels sprouts need to be steamed; salads need to be eaten raw. You can even blend your vegetables (for example, kale) with a few berries or berry-flavored stevia. If you have a thyroid problem and want to eat cruciferous, make sure you add sea kelp for extra iodine, as cruciferous does deplete some iodine.

Now, the biggest point about vegetables is to eat them in large amounts.

Based on your nutritional requirements for vitamins and minerals, vegetables are the best way to get them. Potassium requirements are very high; roughly 4,700 milligrams per day. You would need to consume 7 to 10 cups of salad or vegetables per day to obtain your potassium, and of course if you did this, you would also fulfill your requirements for both vitamins and minerals.

Make sure you avoid MSG in dressings or condiments.

Hunger between meals

I used to advise people to eat five to six small meals per day or have snacks between meals. This was the wrong advice; sorry. The information I somehow missed was that eating, in general, raises insulin. Eating anything raises insulin. Wow, this was new for me, but it was a huge missing piece of the puzzle. This means you should have only three meals per day. If you can eat two meals per day, that would be even better.

The inability to do well between meals due to too great a hunger indicates you are only burning sugar; you are not burning fat. If you crave sugar, you are not burning fat. This all comes from insulin resistance.

If you are not hungry in the morning, then do not eat. This notion that we all need to eat breakfast even if we are not hungry is false information. The idea that someone is not losing weight because they are not eating enough is not true. Listen, if you are not hungry in the morning, it means that your body is eating your belly fat as fuel. Why stop this?

This way of eating is called intermittent fasting. So don't eat between meals.

Consume the right amount of protein for your body type

There is a "sweet spot" for protein: between 3 and 6 ounces per meal. Going too low or too high can affect your blood sugars, digestion and sleep. Also ensure that the quality of protein is good. Soy protein isolate and processed meats are the worst, and organic, grass-fed and pasture-raised meats are the best.

Consume the right amount of fat for your body type

Most people are not consuming enough dietary fat, and I am not talking about deep-fried donuts. Fat with your meals is essential to prevent hunger and snacking and to keep you satisfied. Fat is the only type of food that doesn't spike insulin, as carbs and too much protein will do. Always start gradually, and increase your dietary fats with meals until you feel satisfied and can go between meals without excessive hunger, you experience no cravings, and you have energy between meals.

Avoid gland blockers

Anything containing estrogen will block your glands (especially your thyroid gland). This includes birth-control pills and hormone replacement therapy. Non-organic vegetables contain pesticides, herbicides, insecticides, etc., which also mimic estrogen and can block glands; these are called endocrine disruptors. Too much caffeine can negatively affect your adrenals. Medications can also interfere. If you have to continue your meds, ensure you consume lots of cruciferous foods to counter their effects.

Avoid fluid retainers

Anything with MSG (monosodium glutamate, or modified food starch) will cause fluid retention. MSG has tons of sodium, which is hidden and not even salty tasting. Think about how thirsty you get after eating at a Chinese restaurant or even any fast-food restaurant. Water follows sodium.

MSG also increases insulin up to 300 percent, depending on how much you take. MSG makes you fat.

I am not against your eating sea salt. We all need some salt. We require about 1,000 grams of sodium per day, which is around ¼ teaspoon. The correct thing to do is to add more potassium to counter the excess salt. Potassium works with and partners with sodium. If one goes up, the other goes down. Most people have a sodium excess due to potassium deficiency.

The foods that rid your body of excess fluid are vegetables. Make a kale shake with kale, beet tops and parsley and watch the fluid come right off. You can also juice the rinds of any melons and lose the excess fluid, but that's only to be done on a temporary basis.

Get your sleep

Without sleep, you're not going to lose weight. Sleep is more important than exercise. In fact, you want to adjust your exercise to your sleep. The less sleep, the more you walk; the better your sleep, the more you increase your duration and intensity of exercise.

Sleep is when you burn the most fat. Most sleep problems come from a stressed-out body.

13

Additional Eating Information

So-Called Natural Foods

Simply because a food product says "Natural" on the label, this does not always mean what is implied. There are five things in foods that you should be aware of:

1. *Pesticides, insecticides and other chemical sprays:* Back in the 1930s we started using chemicals to decrease a 20 percent loss of crops. Presently, with the addition of thousands of new chemicals, we still have a 20 percent loss of crops.

2. *Growth hormones:* Farmers use growth hormones for one thing—to make animals grow faster and bigger.

3. *Antibiotics:* Farmers also use antibiotics to make their animals grow larger, but they are used as well to prevent infection and disease. I believe this is the reason for new strains of nearly impossible to kill microbes.

4. *Animal feed containing restaurant grease and animal waste:* Animal waste is recycled into animal feeds and hidden as "protein isolates." The FDA allows each state to regulate how animal waste is processed and recycled back into animal feeds. It is apparently too toxic and expensive for landfills. Restaurant grease is also recycled into animal feeds. Because the waste grease from fast-food restaurants is a health hazard, these establishments are not allowed to drain their used oils and grease through the sewage system. Their cost-effective "solution"

has been to recycle these oils (including harmful hydrogenated oil) and place them back into animal feeds. Animal offal (meaning waste parts from a butchered animal, garbage or rubbish) is also recycled into feeds, which includes blood, guts and feathers.*

5. *Addictive chemicals added to foods:* Many food producers put addictive chemicals in their products as a means of controlling the consumer into continuing to buy and eat their foods. Monosodium glutamate (flavor enhancer) is one of them. MSG doesn't alter the way food tastes; it increases and enhances the sensitivity of taste buds, acting like a drug to excite them. MSG tricks your brain into thinking the food tastes good. It also inhibits the sensation of being satisfied, so you continue to eat. Because of the sodium in monoSODIUM glutamate, water is retained.

Cutting out foods contaminated with antibiotics, pesticides, growth hormones and other chemicals introduced into our mainstream food supply is essential to your weight loss success as well as to your health. Therefore, it is imperative to consume a good portion of organically grown foods. Organic foods are fertilized and grown without the use of toxic chemicals of any kind. It is not always practical to consume 100 percent organic all the time, but if you can eat 50 percent organic, you'll be doing well.

Sugar and Hidden Sugars

Sugar and hidden sugars are at the top of the fat-making-hormone triggers. Very small amounts of these foods will keep you fully out of fat burning for long periods of time. In fact, the fat on your body comes from the hidden sugars, not from the fat you've been eating. Use the substitution chart on the next page to counter these temptations.

---

* *Sources:* Crickenberger and Carawan (1996); Kirby (1999); Research Consortium Sustainable Animal Production (2000).

Substitute Chart

Snacks and Desserts	Substitute
Chocolate	This is an adrenal deficiency. Find a chocolate that has no added sugars. See the end of chapter 18.
Candies	Use sugar-free candy if you need to.
Crackers	Use flax crackers or non-flour crackers.
Flour products (breads, pasta, cereals, cakes, waffles, pancakes, donuts, cookies, etc.)	Use almond flour in the recipes in chapter 18.
Ice cream	Find an ice cream with no added sugar and no artificial sugars. Sugar alcohol sweeteners are okay. I have created a healthy higher-fat, no-added-sugar frozen dessert, without GMOs or hormones (see Resources section); there is also a delicious ice-cream recipe in chapter 18.
Canned fruit with syrup	Canned fruits are loaded with sugars. The substitute would be veggies with some healthy dip.
Flavored yogurt	Unfortunately even plain yogurt has between 6 and 10 grams of sugar per cup. Out of the yogurt family, plain kefir and some Greek yogurt have the lowest sugars. Sour cream, cream cheese and cheese are acceptable.
White sugar	Use non-GMO xylitol, erythritol and stevia.
White rice	Use cauliflower rice. See chapter 18 for recipe.
Oatmeal (prepackaged)	I don't recommend oatmeal. But if you make a granola with seeds and nuts, that would be fine. See chapter 18 for recipe.
Sweet fruits (all fruits, except lemon and limes)	Lemons and limes are great. However, other fruits spike insulin too much and will counter your weight loss.

Gland Blockers

The next chart will give you some substitutes for major gland blockers. Without removing the things that are destroying your endocrine system, it cannot heal.

Gland Blockers	
Avoid	**Substitute**
Alcohol	Non-alcoholic beverages; low-carb light beer is the least damaging—use sparingly
Coffee	Water-processed organic decaffeinated coffee; another option is Teeccino, an herbal coffee, obtainable from health food stores or online at http://www.teeccino.com/
Black tea (caffeinated)	Herb tea or green tea (naturally decaffeinated)
Artificial fats	Real butter, coconut butter (small amounts)
Hydrogenated fats, margarine, Crisco and partially hydrogenated oils	Expeller-pressed oils (small amounts)—coconut, safflower, olive and peanut oils are best to cook with; on salads use flax, olive, sesame seed, sunflower and walnut oils
Deep-fried fats	Deep-fried peanut oil (sparingly)
Commercial eggs (hormone-fed chickens)	Organic pasture-raised eggs
Commercial hamburger, deli meats, pork and chicken	Free-range animal meats, grass-fed or fed on non-GMO, pesticide-free grains and not given antibiotics or growth hormones
Meats with nitrates	Meats without nitrates
Farm-raised fish	Fresh-water or wild-caught fish (hormone-free)
Overcooked beef or steak	Rare or medium-rare steak—fish is an easier-to-digest protein; Liver types do better on less red meat meals (1 to 2 times per week)
Pasteurized milk	Spring water or herb tea
Chips with partially hydrogenated oil (trans fats)	Flax chips

- "Use sparingly" means out of all the foods in this category you could have just one per week; however, it is recommended that you eliminate them altogether. The worse off your metabolism, the less you can get away with the "use sparingly" group.
- Many people think because bread is whole wheat, it is healthier and less fattening. There's not much difference in the speed at which these flour products turn into sugar and then fat. Often commercial whole-wheat bread is exposed to more chemical sprays than white bread because it has more nutrition and so attracts more pests.

Water Retainers

Avoiding water retainers is equally as important as avoiding things that destroy your hormones. You might find it challenging to avoid these high-sodium items, especially when eating out. I've included a helpful chart on the next page.

Beverages

Juices, sodas and soft drinks have high sugar content, and diet sodas and other drinks contain undesirable artificial sweeteners and/or artificial colors. In many areas, tap water isn't the best thing to drink due to the chemicals used to purify the water. Substitute these drinks with those in the right column of the Beverage Substitution Chart below.

Beverage Substitution Chart	
Beverages	**Substitute**
Juices	Unsweetened naturally decaffeinated herb tea, spring water, and water with half a squeezed lemon
Gatorade	Spring water with squeezed lemon; you could also add a hint (1–2 tsp) of apple cider vinegar with 1–2 tsp of lemon to a glass of water to provide extra electrolytes
Tap water with high levels of chlorine	Spring water, filtered water or carbonated mineral water

Water Retainers	
Processed Foods	**Substitute**
Salad dressings with monosodium glutamate (MSG)	Salad dressings without MSG—get the ones with the least chemicals and ingredients; use olive oil and Bragg Liquid Aminos (tastes like soy sauce)
Taco seasoning, repackaged (with autolyzed yeast extract—MSG)	Homemade taco seasoning with onion, sea salt, garlic, chili peppers and paprika
Onion dips, vegetable dips, herb dips and guacamole dips with yeast extract (MSG)	Dips without MSG (go to the local health food store)
Ketchup (commercial)	Sugar-free ketchup
Mayonnaise (commercial)	Mayonnaise from a health food store (365 is a good brand)
Chinese restaurant foods	Homemade Chinese foods with Bragg Liquid Aminos
Rich sauces, like gravies	Sour cream
Spaghetti sauce with sugar/MSG added (especially high-fructose corn syrup)	Spaghetti sauce with minimal sugar added (Muir Glen and Walnut Acres are good brands)
Meats with dextrose sugar or high-fructose corn syrup	Meats containing no sugars (read labels)
Soups with MSG (mostly as autolyzed yeast extract or modified food starch)	Organic soups without MSG
Artificial sweeteners (aspartame and Sweet'N Low)	Stevia, xylitol and erythritol

Recommended Liquids Chart	
Use Most Often	
Herbal tea or green tea	Filtered water
Spring water	Well water
Lemon water	Carbonated water
Use Sparingly	
Rice milk	Organic coffee (one small cup, in the morning)
Almond milk	Milk (if you do, always use organic)

Mercury in Fish

Do not eat shark, swordfish, king mackerel or tilefish, because they contain high levels of mercury. Five of the most commonly eaten fish that are low in mercury are **shrimp, canned light tuna, salmon, pollock and catfish**. Another commonly eaten fish, albacore ("white") tuna, has more mercury than canned light tuna. So, when choosing tuna, purchase the **canned light tuna**.*

Clarification on Protein

Many people have the idea that 6 ounces of meat is 6 ounces of protein. However, these are two different things. No food in nature is pure; foods are always combinations of many factors. For example, let's take one egg. It weighs 56 grams yet has only 7 to 9 grams of protein, 5 grams of fat, 240 milligrams of cholesterol, and 1 gram of carbohydrate. The rest is a compound of minerals, some fiber, etc. So when we talk about foods that are proteins, we are talking about what they are predominately composed of. Nuts, for example, are fat and protein. Beans are mostly carbohydrate and protein. But as we move away from whole foods and into refined foods, we get more concentrated single categories—table sugar being 100 percent carbohydrate.

---

* *Sources:* U.S. Dept. of Health and Human Services and U.S. Environmental Protection Agency (2004).

Protein Amounts		
Amount	**Food**	**Grams of Protein**
1	Egg	7 grams
1	Chicken leg	10 grams
1	Chicken breast	20 grams
3 oz	Small can of tuna	20 grams
3 oz	Sardines (in water)	20 grams
6 oz	Large can of tuna	40 grams
3 oz	Fish	20 grams
6 oz	Fish	40 grams
3 oz	Meat/hamburger	30 grams
3 oz	Turkey meat	20 grams
1 oz	Cheese	7 grams
3 oz (½ cup)	Cottage cheese	15 grams
¼ cup	Nuts/seeds	8 grams
2 Tbsp	Peanut butter	9 grams

The above chart will give you a quick conversion to grams of different food amounts so that you can combine them to equal roughly 25 grams of animal protein per day. Several vegetarian proteins are listed as well. There is also an illustration of these gram amounts on the next page.

Eggs—the Perfect Food

The egg is almost the perfect food for health and weight loss. It is easily digestible as well as a complete food. Eggs give the liver the building blocks it needs to regenerate. Cholesterol levels are not increased by eating them and you can lose weight by including them in your diet. The only time I would avoid eggs is if you have an allergy to them.

Eggs contain ingredients to develop a healthy body, including nearly all of the essential nutrients, such as B_1, B_6, folic acid and B_{12}. They contain the key minerals calcium, magnesium, potassium, zinc and iron. Choline and biotin, which are important for energy and stress reduction, are also found in eggs, and they are complete in all amino acids (protein building blocks).

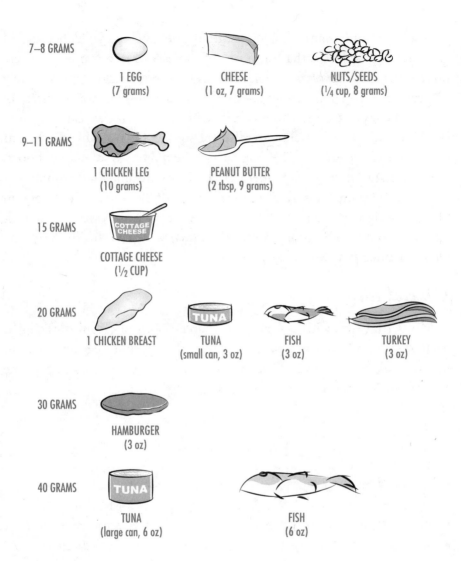

7–8 GRAMS

1 EGG
(7 grams)

CHEESE
(1 oz, 7 grams)

NUTS/SEEDS
(¼ cup, 8 grams)

9–11 GRAMS

1 CHICKEN LEG
(10 grams)

PEANUT BUTTER
(2 tbsp, 9 grams)

15 GRAMS

COTTAGE CHEESE
(½ CUP)

20 GRAMS

1 CHICKEN BREAST

TUNA
(small can, 3 oz)

FISH
(3 oz)

TURKEY
(3 oz)

30 GRAMS

HAMBURGER
(3 oz)

40 GRAMS

TUNA
(large can, 6 oz)

FISH
(6 oz)

The fats in the egg yolk are in close to perfect balance. These essential fats are crucial in the regulation of cholesterol. That is because the antidote to cholesterol is lecithin, which helps dissolve cholesterol, and egg yolks are loaded with lecithin. Make sure not to overcook the yolks, as this will destroy the lecithin. These yolk fats in your diet lower the risk of heart disease. Eggs have almost zero carbohydrates and have the highest rating for complete proteins (containing all the amino acids) of any food. Amino acids are necessary for repairing tissue as well as for making hormones and brain chemicals.

As a side note, many people are afraid of eating egg yolks because of cholesterol. The fact is that most of the cholesterol in our blood is there not because of what we've eaten. Actually, our livers make approximately 75 percent of the cholesterol that exists in our blood. The more cholesterol we eat, the less the body will make. The less cholesterol we eat, the more the body will make. If cholesterol were so bad for us, why would our bodies make so much? The body is an incredible system that knows exactly what to do to create synergy. When we consume foods containing cholesterol, we only absorb 2 to 4 milligrams of cholesterol per kilogram of body weight per day. So, even if we were to eat a dozen eggs each day, we would only absorb 300 milligrams, which is, by the way, the recommended maximum daily amount.

Omelet Ideas

Mix 2 to 3 eggs with sea salt and 2 tablespoons of cream until fluffy. Melt ⅛ stick of butter in a pan over medium heat; pour eggs in pan and lightly cook for 1 minute. Place mixture of fillings on top and flip one side of omelet over until the omelet is slightly browned.

Filling Options

- eggs + goat cheese
- eggs + salsa
- eggs + sautéed mushrooms and onions
- eggs + ground turkey and cheese
- eggs + red peppers and spinach
- eggs + cut tomatoes and green peppers
- eggs + crab and cheese
- eggs + 3 cheeses
- eggs + chicken chunks and cheese
- eggs + avocado slices
- eggs + cream cheese
- eggs + cheese and broccoli
- eggs + meatballs and tomato sauce
- eggs + salmon and cheddar cheese
- eggs + basil leaves and melted cheddar cheese
- eggs + ground beef and Parmesan cheese
- eggs + sun-dried tomatoes with onions and basil leaves
- eggs + tomatoes, mushrooms and onions
- eggs + zucchini and eggplant

14

Sticking to It— GUARANTEED!

Here's the deal. It is highly unlikely that you will stick to this plan without this chapter. I am going to give you some cool ideas to handle certain situations. That's what you've been missing.

I have a lot of experience in overcoming every possible barrier that comes up. So even if you're a stress eater or you attend social events, you'll have solutions that will work.

Temptation

Everywhere you look, it's in your face: ice cream, breads, cookies, cakes . . . SUGAR.

One of my favorite tips is basically replacing your junk with healthy treats that taste the same or better. The recipes in this book will blow you away: chocolate, cookies, candy bars, English muffins, and even ice cream; but of course without the sugar, flour or bad stuff. In addition, chapter 13 is full of ideas for substitute foods.

Stress Eating

What's ironic is that the food people eat to reduce stress actually adds more stress. From sweets they get a spike in blood sugar and an immediate drop. Now they are really stressed out, irritated, grouchy, and craving sweets even more. Eating sweets and refined carbs depletes potassium, calcium and vitamin B$_1$—the three key nutrients to keep your nervous system calm.

Stress tends to keep you from being in the present. When you are not in the present, you do not always think logically or think about consequences. You just want it now and couldn't care less what's going to happen tomorrow.

So here's the technique. Make it okay with yourself to eat that junk food . . . as long as you are fully aware of what you are doing and you are okay with the consequences.

At the very back of this book, I created a cut-out page so that you can tear out the page, then cut out the wallet-size cards and keep them with you. Make it a requirement to read them BEFORE you give in to your temptation. This may discourage you from giving in, especially if you are unwilling to not burn any fat for 72 hours.

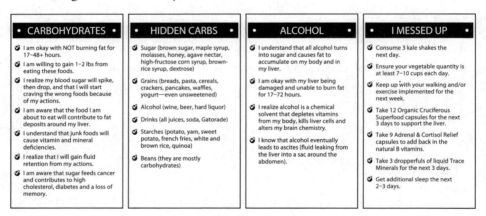

• CARBOHYDRATES •	• HIDDEN CARBS •	• ALCOHOL •	• I MESSED UP •
☑ I am okay with NOT burning fat for 17–48+ hours.	☑ Sugar (brown sugar, maple syrup, molasses, honey, agave nectar, high-fructose corn syrup, brown-rice syrup, dextrose)	☑ I understand that all alcohol turns into sugar and causes fat to accumulate on my body and in my liver.	☑ Consume 3 kale shakes the next day.
☑ I am willing to gain 1–2 lbs from eating these foods.	☑ Grains (breads, pasta, cereals, crackers, pancakes, waffles, yogurt—even unsweetened)	☑ I am okay with my liver being damaged and unable to burn fat for 17–72 hours.	☑ Ensure your vegetable quantity is at least 7–10 cups each day.
☑ I realize my blood sugar will spike, then drop, and that I will start craving the wrong foods because of my actions.	☑ Alcohol (wine, beer, hard liquor)	☑ I realize alcohol is a chemical solvent that depletes vitamins from my body, kills liver cells and alters my brain chemistry.	☑ Keep up with your walking and/or exercise implemented for the next week.
☑ I am aware that the food I am about to eat will contribute to fat deposits around my liver.	☑ Drinks (all juices, soda, Gatorade)		☑ Take 12 Organic Cruciferous Superfood capsules for the next 3 days to support the liver.
☑ I understand that junk foods will cause vitamin and mineral deficiencies.	☑ Starches (potato, yam, sweet potato, french fries, white and brown rice, quinoa)	☑ I know that alcohol eventually leads to ascites (fluid leaking from the liver into a sac around the abdomen).	☑ Take 9 Adrenal & Cortisol Relief capsules to add back in the natural B vitamins.
☑ I realize that I will gain fluid retention from my actions.	☑ Beans (they are mostly carbohydrates)		☑ Take 3 dropperfuls of liquid Trace Minerals for the next 3 days.
☑ I am aware that sugar feeds cancer and contributes to high cholesterol, diabetes and a loss of memory.			☑ Get additional sleep the next 2–3 days.

Discouraged by No Results

There are several points I want to make about no results. The first one is to make sure you are really not getting results. If you base your results on only weight loss, you could be making a mistake. For example, if you are truly getting healthy, your body may have to rebuild body proteins, which are heavier than fat. Gaining muscle mass could give you the false impression that you have stopped losing fat, but in reality the program is working. The best way to know if you are achieving results is to ask: Is your stomach getting smaller? Is your energy improving? and (the big one) Are your cravings disappearing? Focus on achieving these improvements and the weight will eventually come off.

The second thing I teach my clients is to focus on the other related health problems, starting with sleep and stress. Your end weight is the end result of getting healthy; so if things have slowed down, look at all other health problems and focus on whatever is a problem.

Another few points involve foods that may be slowing you down. Are you consuming any hidden sugars? Did you get the point I mentioned earlier about how consuming even tiny amounts of sugar can block fat burning for a few days? Is this happening? Are you snacking between meals? This will keep your insulin too high.

And finally, are some of the new vegetables—like kale—bloating you? If you have bloating, even with healthy foods, you will not lose weight because it's acting as stress. So ensure you do not eat anything that bloats you. Some people have to go real slow on adding fats to their diet.

Craving Sweets

I don't expect you to struggle with cravings while on this plan. If you are doing everything correctly, you will burn fat and you will not burn as much sugar anymore—this means the cravings for sugar will go away. It will take eliminating sugars completely to fully get rid of cravings, because if you leave even a little bit of sugar in the diet, the body will never switch to fat burning. No more sugar cravings is the perfect indicator to let you know you are finally burning fat!

Eating out of Boredom

This is the worst problem. People hate to be bored, and this will get you into trouble with your eating. The only way I know to handle this is to keep yourself busy—real busy. Schedule yourself with more stuff to do so that you don't end up sitting in front of the TV with nothing to do but stick things into your mouth.

Eat Everything on Your Plate?

This has been programmed into us from birth. People are starving around the world, and if you eat all your food, then . . . hmm, not sure what will happen. First of all, so many restaurants put way too much food on the plate. It's actually hard to eat it all. Just eat until you are full and take the rest home. If you are at home, set things up with smaller plates or smaller servings. I know my grandmother just wanted to feed everyone—she lived for it and it meant survival to her. Well, here's the thing: You're not starving; you're not going to starve; there is plenty of food to go around. So, really pay attention to your feeling of satisfaction and just stop eating when you're full. Avoid being stuffed.

Rewarding Yourself with Food

Do you ever reward yourself with food for doing something good? It's an interesting concept. If you really want to reward your body, reward it with a cucumber or a bell pepper—how about that? When you go to Domino's Pizza and the ice-cream shop to reward yourself after a long week of hard work, you're really creating damage to your liver. But I do know that people eat to enhance their mood, and there is incredible sensation with food. So create some healthy substitute foods to replace the junk, and you'll have the same sensation.

Social Situations or Eating Out

There will be a constant distraction with social situations: birthdays, events, universities, holidays, going out with family. Here are a few tips:

- Ensure that you do not go into these situations too hungry—even eat something before you go. The hunger combined with the environment will be rough on your willpower.

- I also make it a personal agreement to get back on track if I go off my plan. The last thing you need is to go off and stay off your plan. I see this with birthday parties a lot. You eat your cake, and the next day, the leftovers; then the following day(s) your blood sugars drop, keeping you searching for more crack . . . I'm sorry, sugar. Realize that it is hard to get into fat burning and very easy to go out of it.

- If you do cheat, then make up for the damage and eat super clean the next day and take an extra supply of your nutrients.

- Tell the host or waiter/waitress to not bring bread to the table or offer dessert.

- If you have an event at your house, add some healthy substitute foods—people will not know the difference, and you control what everyone eats.

- Set a new trend with your family. Get your family and friends to start watching Dr. Berg YouTube videos, and before you know it, the people around you will be more supportive. It's amazing how people will think you're strange for not eating junk foods. They will ask you, "When will you be able to eat normally again?" Really? This IS normal, and we need to start a new trend—actually I need your help to do this.

More Tired on the Plan

When you burn fat and you are in the state of ketosis (fat burning), your body uses more B vitamins. One that it uses is called B_5, or pantothenic acid. There are other B vitamins that also become depleted, such as B_6 and biotin. This is a simple thing to solve—take some nutritional yeast. All you need is one teaspoon per day. You can buy this at a health food store or order a bag on Amazon.com; but try to get non-fortified nutritional yeast, which means no synthetic vitamins are added. The problem is finding a way to consume this powder. You could add it to a shake or mix it with a little peanut or almond butter.

Constipated on the Plan

If you become more constipated on this plan, it could be the additional vegetable fiber. Your gut microbes consume fiber as their food. Adding cruciferous vegetables could overload your microbes and create overwhelm. A simple solution: change some of the vegetables to spinach and use less kale, cabbage or broccoli and see if this handles it. If you need a laxative, the best one to start with is Smooth Move tea (slippery elm bark).

Vivid Dreams

Vivid dreaming and especially nightmares result from a B-vitamin deficiency. Simply add non-fortified nutritional yeast at one teaspoon per day and see the fast change.

15

Body Issues That Interfere with Losing Weight

Forget about focusing on the scale. Weight loss numbers are very misleading. First of all, you could be losing fat and gaining muscle and still be depressed because you're not losing weight. The best indicator that this program is working is that you are getting healthy—more energy, higher stress tolerance, no cravings, good digestion, reduced inflammation, and so on. Remember, the weight is not the problem—it's only the symptom. Refocus on eliminating the real body problems and the weight will come off.

Why?

Because you're never going to lose weight over a tired, stressed-out, bloated, constipated, inflamed, PMSy (if that's a word) body. In this chapter, I will give you some things to improve these "other" body conditions.

The following are the most common body conditions that either interfere with losing weight or indicate a deeper problem:

- Fatigue
- Sleep problems
- Cognitive problems
- Low stress tolerance
- Cravings
- Digestive problems
- Inflammation
- Menstrual and menopause problems

Fatigue

There are several reasons why one is tired. The most common cause is a lack of restful sleep; if this is your problem, go directly to the sleep section. Another cause: tiredness could be related to the thyroid not working. And then you could have blood sugar spikes that create fatigue too. The mistake people make is to try to boost their energy without fixing the real cause of the problem.

If you are sleeping and have decent blood sugar but have a known thyroid problem, study chapter 7.

I have also observed another interesting reason for fatigue that relates to old head trauma or injury. If you have ever been hit in the head, or fell down on your head or face, then later in life developed fatigue, you could be experiencing a physical fatigue in your head from the injury. So I ask people who are tired, "Where is this fatigue located?" And if they say, "In my head area," I ask if they have ever had any trauma in that area. They usually reflect and say something like, "Oh yes, my brother threw a baseball and it hit my head when I was 13."

If this is the case for you, then I have an acupressure injury technique you can use to release and relax the physical stress from the head.

Injury Technique

Here's what you can do: Press either on the opposite side of the head or press into the area of impact, but never directly on the area. Press toward the impact from different angles. See below.

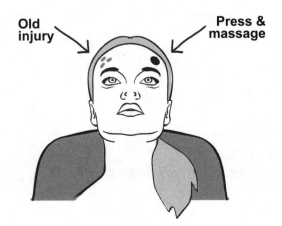

Sleep Problems

This is the most common barrier to losing weight. The most widespread cause of sleep problems is an overactive adrenal gland that is keeping you in stress mode. There are three other causes of sleep difficulties listed below. However, if you suspect adrenal involvement, go to chapter 16 for techniques to reduce stress.

Hot flashes can keep you from sleeping. See page 230 for information on that one.

And an overactive bladder can keep you up all night. Many men with prostate problems have this, and women who go through menopause also have frequent urination while trying to sleep. The eating plan I am recommending will greatly improve this. Why? Because one of the main causes of excessive urination is insulin resistance. Talk to any diabetic—they typically urinate way too often. Wherever the sugar goes, the fluid goes. Just follow the eating plan and you should have a great improvement in holding your urine.

Sleep apnea can also keep you from breathing at night, thus preventing a good night's rest. Some people need oxygen to sleep . . . I know; it's weird, isn't it? If you have sleep apnea, follow the techniques for adrenal stress because this is most likely an adrenal issue. The sinuses enlarge and swell with adrenal stress. Go to chapter 16 for stress-reducing techniques.

Poor Cognitive Function (Memory)

Memory problems nearly always start with an insulin problem. We have talked about this in previous chapters. The prediabetic condition called insulin resistance or hypoglycemia (low blood sugar) is the most common cause. This is because insulin won't let the glucose enter the brain. If your brain starves for fuel, brain cells will die off. Following the eating plan will greatly improve insulin resistance, and you will see positive changes in your cognitive function.

Low Stress Tolerance

This is one of the best indicators for adrenal stress or adrenal fatigue (same thing). The weaker the adrenals, the less you can handle stress. It tends to start off gradually, with just being edgy; then it develops into having the tiniest little thing cause a blowup. It could be something like someone driving too slowly in front of you. Since the adrenals are the stress glands, designed to counter stress states, things people do that show their incompetency or stupidity, their insanities and illogical actions, tend to rub you the wrong way big time. So, in the past they maybe didn't bother you—now they definitely do.

The two powerful things I recommend are a nutritional remedy and a group of stress-reducing acupressure techniques. My adrenal nutritional remedies, which you can find in the Resources section, are designed to address inner stress and nervous tension.

The acupressure techniques for the adrenals are in chapter 16. These techniques can be done with a massage tool or your own hands. The body stores stress in several places. You will use these techniques before bed each night for a wonderful feeling of stress relief. I do them every night before bed. Life gives you stress, and the goal is to release it before you sleep at night.

Cravings for Carbs or Sweets

Cravings are one of the best ways to tell what type of fuel you are burning. You will not crave sweets or carbs IF you are burning fat fuel. It is not normal to crave sweets unless something is out of balance. The problem is that most people do not burn fat due to higher insulin and are forced to live only on sugar fuel. As soon as blood sugar drops too low, following the insulin spike (insulin overreacts to the sugar you ate, pushing blood sugar excessively low), you will be focused on sugar.

The other cause of sugar cravings is insulin resistance. This is a state where your body is blocking insulin, and thus sugar, from entering the cells. Well, insulin is the gatekeeper for other nutrients as well, and if you have insulin resistance, your cells and brain will stay hungry. They will be craving and unsatisfied. Just being on this eating plan will reduce cravings greatly, if not eliminate them.

Inflammation

The main anti-inflammatory hormone in the body is cortisol. We talked about this in the adrenal section. You know that too much cortisol causes belly fat and a whole host of other problems. But having the correct amount of cortisol is essential for life. Cortisol has other functions, which are also used in medicine, and it is made synthetically. Prednisone, cortisone shots or creams, and steroid inhalers are synthetically made cortisol and are all medications used for inflammation, arthritis, asthma, allergies, skin problems of every kind, infections, poison ivy—and the list goes on and on.

Cortisol helps the immune system, the healing process, and the skin; it is a major anti-inflammatory. When you run out of this hormone, you get inflammatory conditions. This is why supporting the adrenals goes a long way in reducing inflammation. The goal is to combine the eating plan, the acupressure techniques, exercise and nutrition to fix your adrenal function so as to get the adrenals to make anti-inflammatory hormones.

There are other reasons for inflammation. I observed that many people who have fibromyalgia happen to have it on the right side of the body. When we support the gallbladder and liver, it all magically disappears. If this is your situation, add the Gallbladder Formula (see Resources section) and use the acupressure Liver Technique provided in chapter 12. Think about it: the remedies most people use for reducing inflammation are actually fats like omega-3 fatty acids, right? Well, if you can't digest them because the gallbladder is sluggish, this could be a barrier in removing pain and inflammation. The gallbladder, if sluggish, can refer pain to the upper right side of the body, neck, head, and even down the arm, hand and fingers on the right side of your body. This is very common. If a person has right-side inflammation and no known injury, then we can suspect gallbladder involvement.

The last reason why someone might have inflammation has to do with high insulin. No worries on this because the recommended eating plan will greatly improve this condition.

Menstrual

If the menstrual cycle is heavy and crampy, then we know your estrogen levels are too high. Estrogen in excess can suppress the thyroid. It can also inhibit bile release and the gallbladder from working. High amounts of estrogen are responsible for hypothyroid conditions. This explains why so many women don't feel better when they take thyroid meds. It also explains why many women develop thyroid problems during and after pregnancy (due to the high levels of estrogen).

To get support for the menstrual cycle, go to the Resources section for further information.

Hot Flashes

Hot flashes can keep you up at night and create a block on losing weight. The root cause of hot flashes is the failure of your adrenals to transition into a state where they back up the ovaries. During menopause, the adrenal glands are supposed to, in theory, take over producing the female hormones once the ovaries go into retirement. But that only happens if the adrenals are strong enough.

If the adrenals are weak going into menopause, hot flashes will usually develop. This symptom shows an inability of the adrenals to produce enough of the right hormones.

There is supportive nutrition that you can take, but I do not recommend going right onto hormones, even if they are natural bioidentical hormones. Anytime you take hormones, the glands that are normally supposed to make hormones become somewhat inactive. It's much better to support the gland than it is to give the body added hormones. See the Resources section for additional information.

16

Ridding Your Body of Stress

D id you realize that all the stress you have ever been exposed to could still be influencing your health? You can equate stress events to adding more applications on your desktop computer. Over time, these stress events drain the adrenals just as more applications slow down your computer. Why? Because the adrenal function is to react and adapt to all stress.

In this section, I want to teach you how to extract stress from the body using my acupressure methods. You will need my massage tool, which I designed to imitate my own hand. Personally, I use it each night before bed to get to sleep and stay asleep.

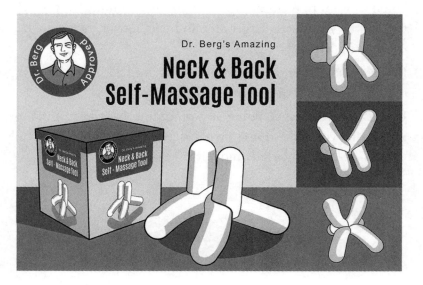

Massage Tool

The acupressure device shown here has three widths: narrow, medium and wide. It's designed so it can be used on people of different sizes.

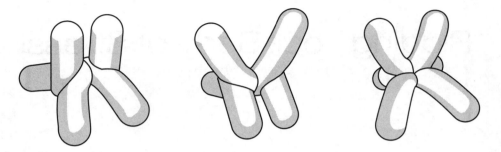

Rules for Use

1. Never press to the point where it feels uncomfortable.

2. All of the techniques you are going to apply should feel good if you have the correct width, correct body point location, and the correct pressure. Since this is a do-it-yourself procedure, it's easy to control how much pressure is used.

3. I recommend covering all seven points each night for 1 minute each. You may want to focus on the neck points 2 minutes longer. Some of the points will cover a larger area and take longer, especially because they have a left and a right side.

4. If you are sore after the techniques, wait until all the soreness is gone before performing the procedure again.

5. If you feel worse after doing any procedure (this is rare), it usually means that your digestion is involved. If this is the case, focus only on the points below the right and left rib cage.

Quick Overview

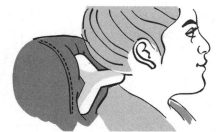

#1 UPPER-NECK POINTS

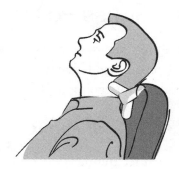

#1 UPPER-NECK POINTS

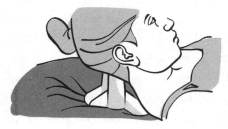

#2 OCCIPITAL POINTS

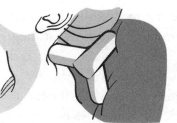

#3 MID-NECK POINTS

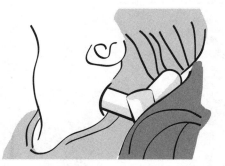

#4 LOWER-NECK POINTS

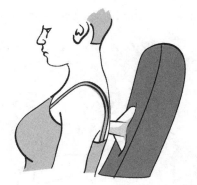

#5 MID-BACK POINTS

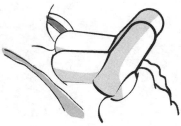

#6 COLLARBONE POINTS

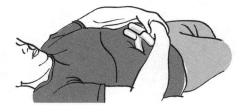

#7 ADRENAL POINTS

The 7 Stress Points

There are seven main areas of your body that hold most of your body's stress. I recommend that you perform the following seven techniques each night before going to bed.

#1 Upper-Neck Points

This first technique is the most important because it extracts the most stress. It's very powerful to ease your stress and enhance your sleep.

Most people use the widest part of the tool for this one, but others may use the medium width. Start by placing the widest part just under the bottom of your skull, at the top of the neck, and lean back.

The best place to do Technique #1 (upper-neck points) is on your couch, as shown in the image below. If you have a high-back office chair, it also is a good setting for use of the tool. I regularly use this tool in my office. It could also be used in your bed with some pillows, but this setup may introduce too much pressure because the entire weight of your head is placed on the tool. Test it out and position your pillow correctly. The person in the image below is using the medium width.

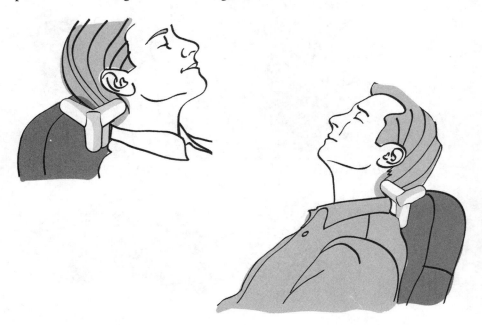

I like to use a couch or a high-back chair for the neck points. Tuck the device just below the skull and let gravity do the work. After 2 to 5 minutes your whole spine will let go and lose tension. The pressure at this location releases the tension down the spine, causing a whole-body relaxation.

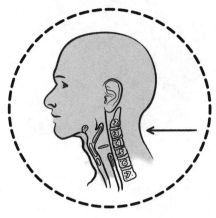

The key is to place the device directly under the back of your skull, where your neck begins (at the first cervical vertebra, which wraps around and overlaps the second vertebra).

Once you position the massage tool, you will find a sweet spot, an area on which it feels good to apply pressure. Let the gravity of your head place pressure on these points (left and right).

How Does It Work?

These points at the top of the neck act as one of the "off" switches of the body. This switch is part of the nervous system called the parasympathetic nervous system or PNS. Another name for the PNS is "rest and digest." These are anti-stress points.

There are even chiropractic techniques that specialize in the first cervical vertebra. This do-it-yourself technique applies low force over 2 to 5 minutes to help align the first segment of your neck. Many people find that once this is perfectly in place the entire spine lines up. The inner connective tissue that protects your spinal cord is called the dura. This dura gets stretched, creating a wonderful relaxation over the entire body.

#2 Occipital Points

The occiput is a bone in the lower back part of your skull.

There are several muscle attachments in this area, and many people feel major tightness here. If you loosen up these upper-neck and occipital muscles, it will feel like you grew an

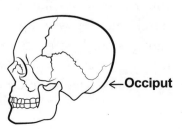

←**Occiput**

inch because your whole spine will be lengthened. On this point, you will use the narrowest part of the massage device and position it at a slightly upward angle, creating some traction, as in the images below.

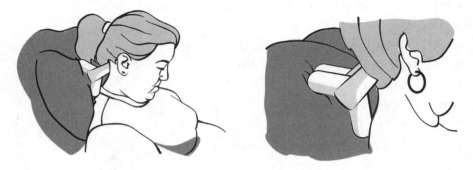

Notice that the head is tilted forward and the device is actually higher (pressing into the skull) than in Technique #1. Let gravity stretch this area; if this is done correctly, you will feel a slight lift to your head.

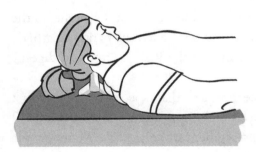

You can also focus on this point while lying down.

Technique #2 is fantastic for people who have had a tailbone injury; when you fall on the tailbone, the force travels all the way up your spine and gets stuck at these points. This technique may also reduce lower-back pain from a tailbone injury.

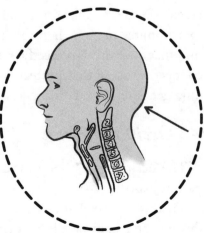

#3 Mid-Neck Points

When you lose the natural curve in your neck and it starts to straighten out—or even worse, exhibit a reversed curvature—lots of tension will occur. This causes the head to feel heavier, as there is no more spring left, and the average head weighs 14 pounds! This technique helps to put the curve back into the neck and removes much of the tension. You will be pressing directly on the middle part of the neck.

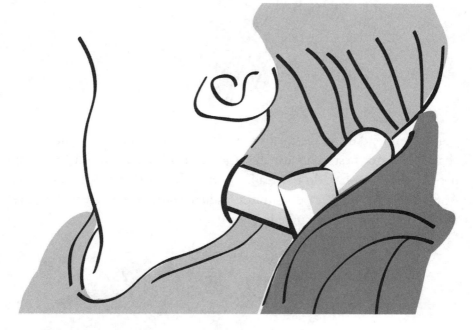

Simply arrange the tool at the mid part of your neck and lie back.

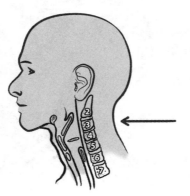

#4 Lower-Neck Points

This is another one with big results. For Technique #4, simply move the device down to the immediately lower part of your neck (C6 area).

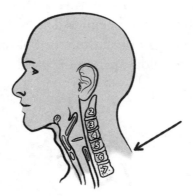

I recommend using the medium width for #4. A couch or a high-back chair will work best. This usually is an area of major tension for many people, yet they often do not realize it until they perform this procedure. Apply pressure for 1 to 2 minutes. When you are done, you'll feel as though you have a nice curve in your neck.

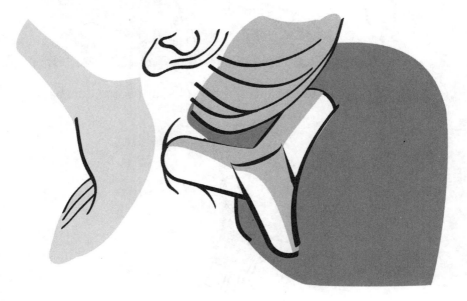

How Does It Work?

This procedure gives people a great deal of relief from accumulated stress, which could include a history of sore throats, whiplash injuries, and tension from sitting in front of a computer for eight hours every day. Pressing inward on these points can provide increased circulation and muscle relaxation.

#5 Mid-Back Points (Static and Dynamic)

Technique #5 is the most difficult to do by yourself; you may need a friend to help you. It can be done on the couch, a high-back chair or your bed, depending on your back sensitivity. Some people feel that using it while lying down provides too much pressure. Use the tripod with the medium points pointed upward.

If you are on your couch, a friend can position and reposition the device at the different areas down the spine. With your friend holding the tool in place, lean back and extend yourself backwards (dynamically). Hold this position for a few seconds. Then have the friend move the massage tool downward on the spine a few inches at a time.

If you are using the tool on your bed, place it in the correct position and then lie back on the device and let gravity do its work statically (without backwards motion). You should hold each new position for 30 seconds at a time. I like to start lower in the mid back and gradually move up every other vertebra. This could give you a tremendous amount of relief, especially if your posture is poor.

You can also do this dynamically by flexing back over the device and then forward. Simply do this several times at each section of your spine as you work downward.

Move the tool down slightly, and then continue to move it all the way down to the bottom of your mid back.

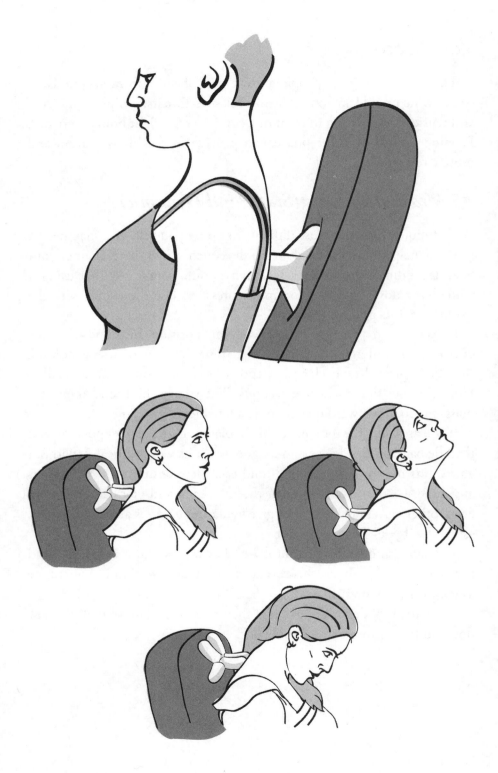

How Does It Work?

The mid back, in an area about one inch to the left and right of the spine, houses the "on" switches of the body. This is the activation part of the nervous system, which is called the fight-or-flight mechanism. Adjust the angle of the tool so it's aligned with the curve of your mid back.

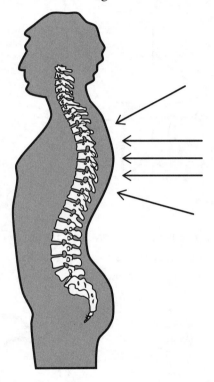

By stimulating these points, you turn off the "on" switch and experience relaxation. You are also reversing your normal forward posture, which facilitates a nice stretch.

#6 Collarbone Points

The muscles under the collarbone are most often ignored. If these muscles are tight (and they usually are), they will cause tension in the neck area and lead to tight upper-back muscles. These muscles become tight after you experience a whiplash injury. Apply the device at different widths under the collarbone and then stretch your neck backwards. This technique will lengthen and stretch the muscles under the collarbone, which will automatically relax your upper-back muscles and loosen your neck—a great exercise to help melt away shoulder tension.

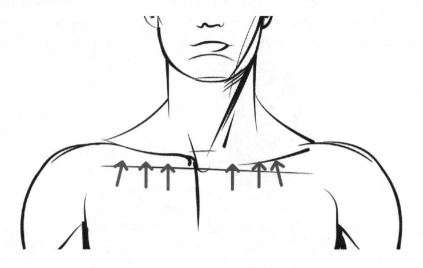

Once you position the tool under the collarbone, you'll want to extend your neck backwards several times as you position the device centrally, then to one side and then the other.

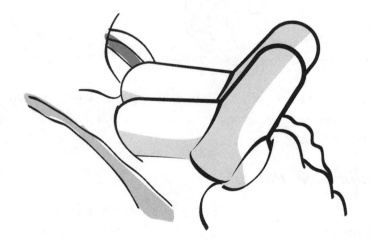

Use the tool to press on the outer parts of your collarbone, both on the left and the right.

#7 Adrenal Points

With this technique, you're not actually pressing on the adrenal gland but on the soft tissue above the adrenals, partly made up of fascia. Fascia is a type of connective tissue, in the form of a sheet or bands beneath the skin, which attaches, stabilizes, encloses and separates muscles and other internal organs. Fascia absorbs stress and tension from the inside of the body and muscles.

Considerable tension can build up within the fascia in your abdomen.

There are several points you'll press to release some of this stress. Make sure you press lightly and gently and apply sustained pressure in this area. There is usually a lot of stress on these points. As seen in the image below, you'll be pressing certain acupressure points, starting on the left side. Press straight down on each point for 30 seconds.

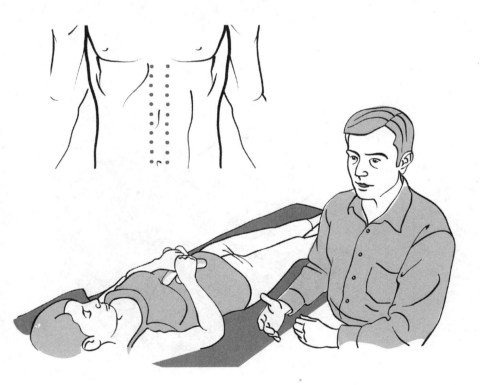

Begin with the left side and press each point on it for 30 seconds, from lower to higher. Then do the same on the right side.

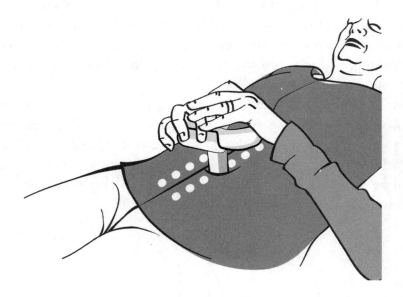

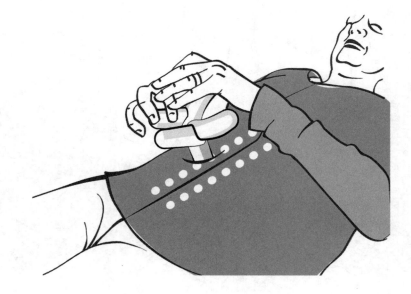

17

Exercising for Your Body Type

Exercising but Still Can't Lose?

You would be shocked to find out how little is known about exercise when it comes to triggering fat-burning hormones. In this chapter, you'll learn the essentials of using exercise as a tool to influence maximum fat burning. You will also discover a new approach that is designed to *burn the most fat* during exercise for your body type and why using the wrong kind of exercise can actually stop weight loss.

There are two principal kinds of exercise: (1) low-intensity, low-pulse-rate endurance exercise, called *aerobic*; (2) higher-intensity, higher-pulse-rate resistance exercise, called *anaerobic*.

If you have an Adrenal body type, you will start with aerobic exercise, because the adrenals are already overworked and putting them into too much stress would make things worse. Overstimulating the adrenals can trigger the stress hormone cortisol, and cortisol can make you fat. With Adrenal types, intense exercise will block the rejuvenation and repair of the body. In some cases, the person will even gain weight with exercise.

Some people with large bellies think they need to just work their abs and the weight will melt off because the abdominal muscles are in the same location as this fat, but that is not how it works. This belly fat is not coming from a lack of exercising of the abdominal muscles; it is coming from the hormone cortisol.

The Ovary body type is a lower-body cellulite fat, which needs a combination of endurance and resistance exercise. Liver and Thyroid body types, on the other hand, respond best to anaerobic (intense) exercise.

However, if you are fatigued, I don't recommend you even start exercising. Let the eating plan build up your energy, and then add in exercise.

Athletes in training, on the other hand, are in a completely different situation and may actually want to train using both aerobic and anaerobic exercise. And for many young people and those who still have their full metabolic systems intact, weight loss may come easily from using either method.

Exercise Doesn't Burn Fat: It Triggers Fat-Burning Hormones to Burn Fat

Exercise is just one of many triggers for fat-burning hormones.

Exercise *n.* a regular series of specific movements designed to stress and activate muscles, causing new cellular adaptations and developments—not merely the burning of calories.

According to this definition, you have to be willing to stress your muscles, which can be uncomfortable.

With a healthy body, the body will very quickly adapt to the stress of exercise, increasing its ability to handle more stress. This is why you have to keep raising the level of difficulty and adding stress in order to continue burning fat.

These physical stresses activate hormones that rebuild and make the body's tissues more able to adapt to new stresses. This requires changes in cellular structures—new enzymes, new capillaries, new mitochondria and larger muscle fibers; and when the body is rebuilding during the rest phase (down time), it uses fat as energy to allow this to occur.

The problem lies with the body's dislike of stress; it has a tendency to want to avoid stress—especially the stress of exercise, since it is uncomfortable pushing through the phases of adaptation. However, to stay in fat burning, you have to continue to make exercise uncomfortable. As soon as you become accustomed to the routine, fat burning stops because the hormones have adapted.

Basic Principles of Exercise and Hormones

There are two basic ways a person could exercise and many variations in between. You could keep the intensity low and exercise for a long time; you could also increase the intensity and exercise for very little time. Each action affects hormones differently.

From a hormone point of view, to create the maximum fat burning you would be better off exercising at high intensity for short time periods with lots of rest in between. This would cause the body to release growth hormone and glucagon,[1] both fat burners. Intense exercise brings about more destruction to the body, influencing hormones to take repair energy from fat. So you are actually destroying the body in order to trigger these hormones to repair and regrow muscle tissue. What's interesting to note is that fat-burning hormones do their work in the rest periods after, *not during*, exercise.

But here's the problem.

If the person is already stressed and their adrenal glands are burnt out, intense exercise can overwhelm the body, creating more damage. This is because of the destructive actions of the hormone cortisol, which tears down muscle tissue, as compared to growth hormone, which builds muscle tissue.

So the Adrenal type's only option is to do low-intensity exercise of longer duration, at least at first. This will cause less stress on the body and it won't take nearly as long to recover. You will trigger some fat burning, but only after 20 to 30 minutes. Most people could even do this daily. However, I would recommend doing it every other day to begin and gradually increasing to daily if possible. This type of exercise is a great way to counter body stress.

Stress in general is regulated by the adrenals. You might have heard about "fight or flight." Well, this is the adrenals' way of reacting to stress. The main hormone triggered is adrenaline; this releases large amounts of stored sugar for quick energy, since the body doesn't have time to burn fat, as it's just too slow. The weaker the adrenals are when going into this program, the less stress you want to experience. Hard-core, intense-type exercise will only irritate the adrenals and release more sugar, not fat. Slow, gentle endurance-type exercise will ease this stress and allow the body to burn more fat and less sugar over time. The goal is to exercise appropriately so as to trigger fat burning and avoid excess stress and sugar burning.

Based on the Body Type Quiz in chapter 4, you will discover what to do first. Those people who have adrenal weakness should start with the low-intensity and then gradually add the higher-intensity exercise.

Calories and Muscle Mass

Calories are units of energy in food.

There is another "popular" idea that building more muscle mass (through anaerobic exercise) will cause the body to burn more calories. This is absolutely true; *however*, what is the source of those calories being burned? Are they from sugar or fat?

Burning calories by building greater muscle mass does not automatically mean that they will come from *fat* calories. When dealing with weight loss, we have to be more concerned with the *type* of calories being burned than with the quantity. When it comes to fat burning, the size of your muscles is insignificant. Look at a football player who has lots of muscle mass yet has lots of fat too. Having large muscles doesn't automatically cause your body to burn more fat.

The most important point to know is that the fat-burning-hormone effect occurs 14 to 48 hours after exercising, BUT only if certain factors are present: adequate sleep, good nutrition, low sugar, low stress and healthy glands.

The following hidden barriers will prevent weight loss:

1. Sleeping less than 7 quality hours. *Quality* means having good deep sleep and feeling rejuvenated.
2. Not resting enough between exercise sessions.
3. Not resting long enough between the repetitions or intense bouts of exercise.
4. Exercising intensely for too long. Intense anaerobic exercise should be kept between 25 and 40 minutes, and even that should include within the workout a good amount of rest between bouts of exercise.
5. Consuming sugars, starches, juice, sports drinks or alcohol. Most protein bars have tons of sugar.
6. Having pain or inflammation.
7. Lots of stress.

Calories Are Insignificant Compared to Hormones

Think about this—if you exercise moderately for one hour, you might burn 350 calories. That's equivalent to several teaspoons of salad dressing. No big deal!

The real benefits of exercise occur one to two days later, but *only* if the environment is almost perfect. In other words, if you do things correctly and don't violate the fat-burning environment, you will burn fat. Fat-storing hormones can easily nullify the fat-burning hormones. The worse off your hormone health, the more perfect the other factors need to be.

Eating Before, During or After

I don't want you to eat before, during or after you exercise. Why? Because adding food will increase insulin and stop weight loss. Keep your meals standard and include exercise where you can do it. The only exception: if you do a massive workout where you feel like your blood sugars have dropped. In this case, add a little protein. But for most people, avoid snacks.

There are people who do long-distance running and they need to have some carbs to continue. I am not going to address or recommend anything for such a case because that is outside the scope of this book.

Rest between Exercises

Rest is crucial between periods of exercise because this is when the body needs energy from the fat to repair itself. You should never exercise over a healing sore muscle. Sore means healing. In most cases, the longer the soreness lasts, the worse off the adrenals. If before the workout you take a teaspoon of flax oil or 3 flaxseed-oil perles (omega-3), this will increase oxygen and speed up the elimination of soreness.

Sleep Quality and Amount

Insufficient sleep will add stress and keep you from burning fat. One goes through four levels of sleep at night, and it's during deep, rejuvenating sleep that fat-burning hormones take effect, especially within the first few hours. Superficial sleep hinders fat burning.

Stress Level

Stress activates cortisol, which has a fat-storing effect. This includes childbirth, divorce, loss of a loved one, pain and inflammation, injury, bad news, work, finances, traffic, and so on.

When losing weight, you should try to maintain a lower stress level. If you find your stress level can't be lowered, you would need to exercise longer—aerobically (light endurance-type).

The Difference between the Body's Two Main Energy Systems

The body, like a machine, needs energy to operate. This requires some type of fuel, in this case food in the form of protein, carbohydrates and fat, which is burned off into energy. You also have stored fuel—sugar and fat.

There are two energy-producing systems in the body that allow us to be in motion. One is for brief high-intensity activity and the other is for low-intensity endurance-type (or long and slow) activity. Under certain circumstances, such as in emergencies or times of sudden intense exertion, we need quick, explosive energy for a short duration. On other occasions, we need longer-lasting endurance-type energy to keep us going for extended periods.

The Aerobic Energy System

Low Intensity—Longer Duration

Aerobic means *with oxygen*. For our purposes here, the aerobic energy system can be defined as burning fuel with oxygen. Your body burns stored fats and stored sugar in the presence of oxygen. An automobile uses a mixture of gasoline and oxygen as its fuel. Similarly, when the body is in the aerobic mode, it uses oxygen in the mixture as well. The aerobic system runs at a turtle's pace—slow to moderate. The heart rate, on average, is between 127 and 130 beats per minute (bpm); however, a better indicator for aerobic exercise is how the person is breathing. A simple way of knowing when you are in the aerobic energy-burning state is that you will be able to speak without the need to take gasping breaths during sentences. In other words, you won't be huffing and puffing for air. With this system, *you begin to burn fat after 30 minutes of exercise*, after burning off the body's "limited" sugar supply.

There are several negative things you can do to nullify the benefits of aerobic exercise, as can be seen in the diagram below. The upper line represents the total amount of exercise, while the lighter lower line represents the *actual benefit* after subtracting things like poor sleep, high stress and/or the wrong foods. For example, on January 4 the person worked out for about 100 minutes, but because of what they ate or because they didn't sleep or had too much stress, the actual benefit was zero.

TOTAL AEROBIC EXERCISE MINUS NEGATIVE FACTORS THAT INHIBIT THE BENEFITS OF EXERCISE

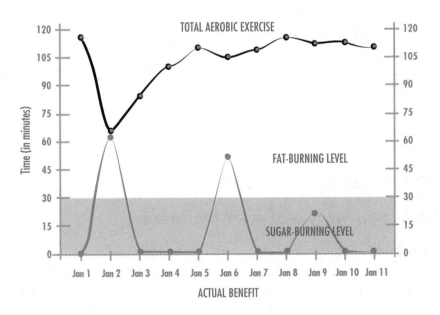

The aerobic energy system is involved in burning fat fuel *during* exercise and slightly after. The other type of exercise, which will be covered in the next section, burns fat *after* bouts of exercise.

Examples of low to moderate activity that would utilize the aerobic energy system include walking, mild treadmill, biking, light jogging, light swimming, light cross-country skiing, and other activities where the required heart rate is maintained.

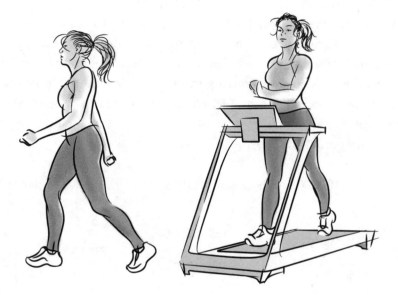

SLOW-PULSE-RATE EXERCISE   MILD TREADMILL

The Anaerobic Energy System

Higher Intensity—Shorter Duration

Anaerobic means *without oxygen*. The anaerobic energy system produces energy without utilizing oxygen; its ONLY source of fuel during the time of exercise is sugar in the blood or stored sugar in the muscles and liver. **This system does NOT initially burn fat fuel during the time you are working out. However, it does stimulate fat-burning hormones 14 to 48 hours later.**[2] (The aerobic system burns fat *during* exercise.) The anaerobic system is used for quick high-intensity exercise and kicks in immediately during exercise when the supply of oxygen becomes inadequate for the activity. Anaerobic gets activated at a higher pulse rate, around 145 beats per minute or greater. It can even get activated with a slow pulse rate if the intensity is high enough.

Some examples of intense exercise that use the anaerobic energy system include running, fast jogging, fast treadmill, soccer, hockey, basketball, swing dancing, wrestling, weight training, sprinting and boxing. It can also include activities such as bike riding and swimming, if the activity is done intensely to the point where the necessary higher heart rate is achieved.

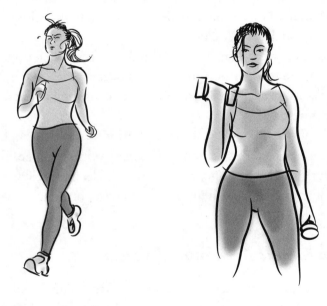

HIGH-PULSE-RATE EXERCISE   RESISTANCE-TYPE EXERCISE

Liver/Thyroid Body Type Exercise Plan

Use Anaerobic Only

The fat-burning hormones are stimulated by *intense* exercise. Anaerobic exercise is intense. The more intense it is, the greater the triggering of fat-burning hormones.

The Benefits of Anaerobic Exercise

Even though this system uses *primarily sugar as fuel during exercise (NOT fat)*, it can help stimulate fat burning because of the fat-burning-hormone effects 14 to 48 hours later. It is delayed. But here's the catch—this only occurs if sugar intake and overall stress are low enough and sleep quality and quantity are sufficient. Many people have wasted tremendous amounts of time and energy with very little result simply by not knowing the above facts. They either attempt to use exercise for the wrong body type or self-sabotage by countering the exercise with nullifiers. If you have an Adrenal body type and do intense or high-pulse-rate exercise, you will not usually lose weight.

Another benefit of anaerobic exercise is the triggering of growth hormone. More growth hormone means deeper sleep. Many people get a better-quality sleep with anaerobic exercise, as long as they don't work out just before bed.

Growth hormone is the anti-aging hormone, and through anaerobic exercise one can keep this hormone within an optimal range. Testosterone also follows growth hormone, which enhances lean muscle mass. Overall, one will burn more fat with anaerobic exercise, but remember there is a day or two delay.

Caution about Anaerobic Exercise

With high-intensity exercise also comes stress. Any stress triggers the hormone cortisol, which can counter the fat-burning hormones. The trick is to exercise intensely enough to trigger fat-burning hormones, yet at the same time keep cortisol (fat-making hormone) low. You accomplish this by SHORT INTENSE BOUTS OF EXERCISE with LOTS OF REST IN BETWEEN. This way the muscles will be activated without stressing the adrenals too much. Overtraining will defeat the entire goal. Once you activate the fat-burning hormones, you can sit back and let them do their job. Make sure you are getting enough rest between exercise periods as well as keeping any and all sugars nil. These are small but important points.

The Hormone Connection to Exercise

To use exercise to trigger fat-burning hormones, it is important to discuss the variables of exercise:

1. Intensity (the power behind the exercise) and difficulty

2. Frequency

3. Duration (total time of exercise)

4. Type

5. Rest

The goal is to use exercise strategically to maximize and keep your body in fat burning and minimize fat-making stress hormones.

Intensity and Difficulty

Intensity is a primary factor; it is the most powerful stimulus for the fat-burning hormones. Growth hormone is the best example of this. If the exercise is not intense enough, you won't be able to stimulate growth hormone.

At the beginning of this exercise program you will stimulate these hormones to burn fat. The body will repair itself and get used to it. The more you get used to the difficulty, the less the fat-burning hormones are affected. So, with time, there will need to be a progressive increase of intensity to create the same effects on fat-burning hormones. You have to keep the difficulty level high in order to keep the intensity high enough. Therefore, you need to keep challenging yourself.

I personally started out biking around my neighborhood on flat pavement. I used to ride my bike through some trails and initially could barely make it up a steep hill—this was intense. Several years later, I am going up very steep hills, which I never thought I could achieve, and it's not even a challenge. So I've had to set my gears lower to make it very difficult going up the hill in order to keep the intensity high. This way I can stay in fat-burning mode. The body adapts and you need to keep challenging it.

Frequency

There are two different frequencies we are talking about. The first is the frequency of repetitions of exercise during one session. The second is how many days per week one exercises.

It is important to keep your workouts short and intense. For anaerobic exercise the repetitions don't have to be many, because as you increase intensity, adding lots of repetitions will also trigger the adrenal stress hormone cortisol and defeat the purpose. If you are doing weight training, instead of increasing repetitions add more weight to increase intensity, but keep the duration short. In the beginning, you'll start out with five repetitions and progress from there. The thing to *not* do is use light weights with a high number of repetitions, as there's not enough intensity to trigger fat-burning hormones.

Anaerobic exercise should be done every other day—not daily—unless you are still sore, in which case you should wait till most of the soreness goes away before working out again. Take more rest between exercises and keep soreness at the low end.

Duration

The actual duration of exercise is also key. If you are being intense and doing it for a long time, you will automatically nullify fat-burning hormones by again stressing the adrenals to pump out cortisol. It's better to keep the intensity high and the duration short and quick. Intense bursts of repetitions for short periods of time, starting at one minute, are best. It is vital to rest for about five minutes between these bouts.

Types of Exercise

There are two main types of exercise with anaerobic:

1. Weight training or resistance training
2. Increased pulse rate

Since the key to stimulating fat-burning hormones is *intensity*, it is best to find the exercise that will give you the most intensity based on your capabilities. If your body doesn't allow you to do hockey, you might want to stick with either doing weight training or using a resistance machine at the gym, where you could get good intense exercise.

Rest and Recovery

This is the most important variable, as the fat-burning hormones are using up fat during the rest between exercises and up to two days after exercise. Without resting, you get very little fat burning.

With some people, an extra 30 minutes of sleep per night as well as reducing their exercise routine to twice or even once per week, with lots of rest in between, will cause them to start burning more fat.

Plateau

The body adapts to the stress of exercise within two to three weeks. It then takes another two weeks to stabilize these tiny body cell structures. This is why people tend to plateau when attempting to lose weight or when starting any exercise program. This is also why it is crucial to change your exercise routines, keeping them new. I recommend rotating their sequence every two to three weeks. That way your body will never get fully accustomed to the routine and your difficulty and intensity will remain high. This is the most important key to staying in fat burning and getting more out of your exercise. Examples of different types of exercise that can be switched would be biking, step aerobics, running, Curves routines, weight training, yoga, boxing routines, rollerblading, racquetball and swimming. The exception is the Adrenal body type, for which you would want to keep the intensity lower and keep the stress of exercise also on the low side. If you have an Adrenal body type, you would focus on aerobic exercise until your adrenals are stronger, then graduate to higher-intensity-type exercise.

Hormones Triggered by Anaerobic Exercise

The first one is **growth hormone**. Remember that this is the anti-aging, fat-burning, lean-body-mass-producing hormone, which also helps prevent the breakdown of proteins—like your bones, muscles, hair, skin and nails. It is stimulated by intense exercise (anaerobic) only. This hormone works through the liver.

The second one is **glucagon**. This is the opposing hormone to insulin, which gives the cells fuel between meals and is also fat-burning. It too works through the liver and is stimulated only by intense exercise.

The third one is **testosterone**. This hormone is made by the adrenal glands, testicles, and even the ovaries. It is a fat-burning hormone in that it is involved in making muscle, as well as giving male characteristics and sex drive in males and females. It follows growth hormone—wherever growth hormone goes, so goes testosterone.

The fourth one is **adrenaline**. This is an adrenal hormone and is the main hormone to release fat energy from the fat cells. It is triggered by stress, such as intense exercise.

The above four hormones have something in common—they all work through the liver. In fact, all fat-burning hormones work through the liver. The better the liver works, the better these hormones work. It's interesting that as the liver improves, body proteins improve too, including hair, nails and skin. That is because of the liver's increased ability to process more growth hormone, which prevents the breakdown of protein in hair, nails, etc. Now this hormone can help manufacture body proteins more efficiently.

Growth hormone and glucagon are triggered not only by exercise but by consuming dietary protein; however, it has to be the correct amount, as excess protein can turn into fat. The weaker the liver, the less protein the person can handle. So if you fix the liver first, the person can tolerate more protein in the diet and thus get more stimulation of these two fat-burning hormones.

Many people go on a high-protein diet and lose weight for two weeks, then the weight loss stops. This is mainly due to a weakened liver, which cannot break down protein efficiently. They might even show signs of protein deficiency, because the liver is blocking the absorption.

The following chart gives you an idea of when fat-burning hormones are triggered in relation to exercise. The trick is to keep cortisol as low as possible yet at the same time keep the others as high as possible.

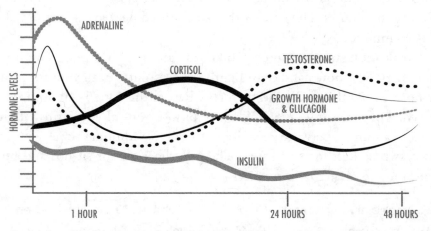

Adapted with permission from Faigin, *Natural Hormonal Enhancement*, 265.

Anaerobic Exercise Routine

1. Keep the intensity high.
2. Do short repetitions of intense exercise, starting at 1 minute.
3. Rest a good amount after each bout of exercise. For example, if you exercise for 1 minute, spend 5 minutes resting afterwards.
4. Exercise between 25 and 40 minutes, but no longer than 45 minutes. This way cortisol will not be raised too high.
5. Exercise every other day with rest between sessions. Do not work out daily.
6. Do not do the entire body; do upper body one day and lower body the next.

Workout example: If you are doing pull-downs on the weight machine, find the weight that is intense enough where you could do 5–7 repetitions. It might take you 30 seconds. Rest for 1 minute. Repeat this 4 times and then rest for 5 minutes. Next, go to bench press and do the same thing. After that, you might want to do rowing, following the same procedure, for 25–40 minutes in all; then you're done.

Workout example: Find how much weight you could squat with, and do 5–7 repetitions. Repeat this 3 times, resting momentarily between reps. After that, rest for 5 minutes. Do the same for hamstrings (back part of the thigh muscle), then leg extensions, for a total of 25–40 minutes.

Workout example: You can do the stationary bike exercise. Get your pulse rate up to 150–180 until your legs fatigue, right around 1–2 minutes. Rest for 5 minutes. Then repeat the same procedure. Do this for a total of 25–40 minutes.

Workout example: Go on a bike ride and get your pulse rate up to 160, then slow down and coast lightly for 5 minutes until your breathing is normal. Do this again and then rest. Repeat this for 25–40 minutes.

Workout example: Do 3–4 sets of push-ups until your arms fatigue, resting a minute between reps. Repeat these 2 additional times with rest in between. Rest for 5 minutes. Then do the same for sit-ups and pull-ups, for a total of 25–40 minutes.

Examples of Anaerobic	Time	Intensity	Difficulty	Soreness
Weight training	25–40 min.	High	Moderate to high	Low
Exercise machine (gym)—resistance	25–40 min.	High	Moderate to high	Low
Home exercise—resistance	25–40 min.	High	Moderate to high	Low
Running	25–40 min.	High	Moderate to high	Low
Sprints	25–40 min.	High	Moderate to high	Low
Sports (basketball, soccer, football, boxing, etc.)	25–40 min.	High	Moderate to high	Low
Biking	25–40 min.	High	Moderate to high	Low
Hiking	25–40 min.	High	Moderate to high	Low
Swing or jazz dancing	25–40 min.	High	Moderate to high	Low
Swimming	25–40 min.	High	Moderate to high	Low
Aerobic dance class	25–40 min.	High	Moderate to high	Low

Anaerobic Exercise Times and Rest Periods						
Week	Mon.	Tues.	Wed.	Thurs.	Fri.	Sat./Sun.	Weekly
1	15 min.	REST	15 min.	REST	15 min.	REST	45 min.
2	20 min.	REST	20 min.	REST	20 min.	REST	60 min.
3	30 min.	REST	30 min.	REST	30 min.	REST	90 min.
4	35 min.	REST	35 min.	REST	35 min.	REST	105 min.
5	40 min.	REST	40 min.	REST	40 min.	REST	120 min.
6	40 min.	REST	40 min.	REST	40 min.	REST	120 min.
7	40 min.	REST	40 min.	REST	40 min.	REST	120 min.
8	40 min.	REST	40 min.	REST	40 min.	REST	120 min.

The first chart, on page 260, shows the factors you should put attention on in anaerobic exercise. The time should be between 25 and 40 minutes, not to exceed 45 minutes. You need enough intense exercise to trigger growth hormone yet not so much that it overstimulates cortisol, which tends to nullify growth hormone. The intensity should be high; on a scale from low to high, you should aim toward high. However, after a while the intensity is relative from person to person, so this needs to continue to increase over time. This also applies to the overall difficulty level (again a relative term from person to person). You should keep it at a moderate to high difficulty level. If it's too easy, fat-burning hormones are not triggered. There is no problem with getting sore after you work out, but you should rest until most of the soreness goes away. In other words, you don't want to exercise over lots of soreness, as you haven't given your body a chance to heal through hormone influences. Also, the adrenal hormone cortisol is activated by soreness and inflammation, so keeping this hormone to a minimum is important.

Keep your anaerobic exercise between 25 and 40 minutes and continue to raise your difficulty level higher over time as your body adapts to the stress you put on it.

The soreness factor is the indicator as to whether or not you should increase the difficulty level. More soreness means hold off and give it more time and more rest. Less soreness means increase the difficulty and intensity.

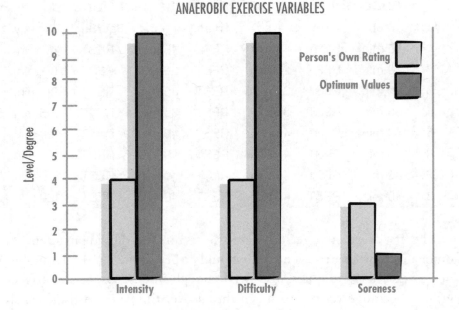

In the following graph, the vertical dark gray bar indicates optimum anaerobic exercise, while the light-colored bar to the right shows the way in which stress, lack of quality sleep and refined carbohydrates nullify exercise.

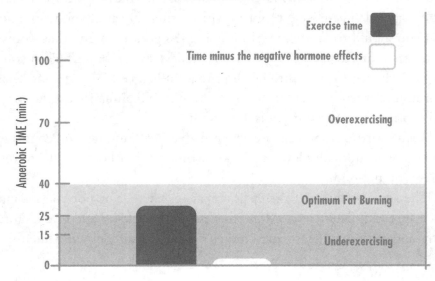

Adrenal Body Type Exercise Plan

Use Aerobic

If the stress gland is stressed, you want to avoid intense exercise. To improve the stress gland, the correct exercise is calming and less stressful. This type of exercise will burn fat mostly during and slightly after the exercise.

The Benefits of Aerobic Exercise

The main benefit of light endurance-type exercise is that it is very gentle on the adrenals and will keep stress hormones to a minimum. However, aerobic exercise doesn't burn fat 14 to 48 hours after exercise like the anaerobic system does.

The problem with anaerobic exercise is that it can stress the adrenals more than aerobic exercise. More intense exercise and exercise that generates a higher pulse rate triggers the stress part of the nervous system—the "sympathetic nervous system"—which monitors the body's fight-or-flight response. As soon as the body goes into this mode, the stress hormones cortisol and adrenaline kick in. If the adrenals are already overwhelmed, cortisol can become excessive for longer periods of time. This will prevent deep sleep and keep the person in a state of nervous anxiety. Cortisol is also the hormone that produces weight gain in the midsection.

Another positive aspect worth mentioning about the aerobic energy system is that its waste products (carbon dioxide and water) are harmless compared to the waste product from anaerobic exercise (lactic acid). Its only drawback, if you looked hard to find one, is it requires time (at least 20 to 30 minutes of slow exercise with the heart rate between 127 and 130 beats per minute) for the body to even *begin* to burn fat.

Working Harder Will Initially Slow Your Progress

Many people think that to melt a lot of dense fat you need a tremendous amount of intense, hard exercise. This is not true. You can burn fat using only light exercise with little effort. You burn fat while you're barely breathing!

In nearly every patient seminar, I've found that the majority of people who are not losing weight with exercise are mixing weight training into their programs. This is a big mistake if they have an adrenal weakness! Weight training is anaerobic and worsens the adrenal glands.

You can see from the chart below the benefits of spending more time doing aerobic exercise. The goal in following this program is to get your body to burn only fat, not sugar. The anaerobic system is working to a small degree during aerobic exercise. But notice what happens to the anaerobic system at 30 minutes; it really shuts down. This is where most people stop exercising—the exact point where the fat burning really begins.

You can also see that if you continue to exercise after the 30-minute point, fat begins to be the predominant fuel; there is great efficiency from this point forward when continuing with aerobic exercise.

Sugar-Burning to Fat-Burning Ratios based on time of aerobic exercise		
Workout Times (min.)	% Sugar Burning	% Fat Burning
1	70	30
2	50	50
4	35	65
10	15	85
30	5	95
60	2	98
120	1	99
> 120	< 1	> 99

Aerobic Exercise Routine

1. Keep the intensity low. Keep it light enough so you can breathe comfortably.
2. Start with 15 minutes per day and work up to 60 minutes per day. (Some people will find they can do more than 60 minutes, but the exercise period should be no longer than 120 minutes per day.) Over time you will get used to this and your body will plateau. When that happens, you could add in the anaerobic exercise.

3. Exercise every other day at first with rest in between. After two months, you could progress to daily.

4. If your body is sore, wait until the soreness goes away before working out again. It is important that your body heal between sessions, as this means your fat-burning hormones are also working.

With Adrenal types, you have to grow back the muscle you have lost from overactive adrenal glands. Since muscle weighs more than fat, you might not initially lose weight but should feel your clothes getting looser. The weight starts dropping two to three months later in some cases.

Examples of Aerobic	Workout Times
Walking	60 min.
Light jogging	30 min.
Biking	60 min.
Treadmill	60 min.
Elliptical machine	60 min.
Swimming	60 min.
Yoga	60 min.

Aerobic Exercise Times and Rest Periods							
Week	Mon.	Tues.	Wed.	Thurs.	Fri.	Sat./Sun.	Weekly
1	15 min.	REST	15 min.	REST	15 min.	REST	45 min.
2	20 min.	REST	20 min.	REST	20 min.	REST	1 hr.
3	30 min.	REST	30 min.	REST	30 min.	REST	90 min.
4	40 min.	REST	40 min.	REST	40 min.	REST	2 hrs.
5	50 min.	REST	50 min.	REST	50 min.	REST	2.5 hrs.
6	60 min.	REST	60 min.	REST	60 min.	REST	3 hrs.
7	60 min.	REST	60 min.	REST	60 min.	REST	3 hrs.
8	60 min.	REST	60 min.	REST	60 min.	REST	3 hrs.

As you can see in the second chart on page 265, a gradual progression is best. In the beginning you might not start burning fat because you are working out less than 30 minutes. But it's recommended that you do this, especially if you are not used to it.

If you keep working out for 30 minutes aerobically, you will never burn fat, since fat burning only starts after 30 minutes. It is also recommended that you don't exercise over an hour, since this can stress the adrenals even more. Exercising up to an hour is a safe bet. Once the adrenals are strong, which could take 8 to 12 weeks, you could then add in the anaerobic exercise.

At this point in the program your body will have enough strength to stay in the aerobic mode, and a combination of both types—aerobic and anaerobic—will keep you from adapting to just one form of exercise. As a person gets used to an exercise and it is no longer difficult, fat-burning hormones will cease to be stimulated; so you need to continue varying it and using different muscles, making it more difficult over time.

Don't Stop Before You Start Burning Fat

Based on surveys of people who could not lose weight with exercise, besides those who were mixing anaerobic with aerobic exercise there were many who used only aerobic exercise, but they did not do it *long enough* to tap into the fat reserves. In order to get the real benefits of the aerobic energy system, you must exercise long enough—60 minutes. If you do this, the results will be great.

History of Long-Term Sugar Consumption

If a person has regularly consumed a lot of sugar for some time, it could take even longer to begin burning fat. Even if they were to exercise aerobically, it might take 40 to 50 minutes or more instead of 20 to 30 minutes to start burning fat. This is because their body's sugar reserves have adapted to a larger reserve storage system. You simply need to eliminate sugars completely, and over a few months the body will adapt back to normal sugar supply levels.

Once your body heals, you will be able to add further anaerobic exercise to your program. Anaerobic exercise actually burns more fat than aerobic, but 14 to 48 hours later; yet if your body is in stress mode, it can only tolerate aerobic exercise at first. Using both systems correctly would be the most optimum.

Ovary Body Type Exercise Plan

Use Aerobic and Anaerobic

If you have an Ovary body type, you need to combine BOTH aerobic and anaerobic exercise. You should do this by exercising every day with anaerobic and either every other day or even daily with aerobic.

The type of fat the Ovary body type has is a superficial cellulite. It is mostly below the bellybutton. So the best type of exercise is lower body—walking, running, treadmill, soccer, basketball, jazz dancing, step aerobics, etc. Focus on working the muscles of the hips, thighs and buttocks. Force these muscles to use energy from the surrounding fat layer. The key with the Ovary body type is intensity, really ripping those muscles hard core. This body type needs the most intensity.

Keeping estrogen low is also essential to getting the weight off. This means consuming foods that are anti-estrogenic—cruciferous vegetables. It also means avoiding growth hormones (mostly estrogen) in the food supply. I would recommend avoiding soy as well, since soy has plant estrogenic qualities.

Summary

Fat is *potential energy*. Fat has enough potential energy to allow a lean person to run 800 miles or last 90 days without food. But most people, with the exception of long-distance runners, never learn how to tap into this amazing potential. Have you ever noticed that long-distance runners are very thin? This is because they normally remain in the aerobic mode when they run and therefore burn fat as their primary fuel.

Some people (especially Adrenal body types) are initially too unhealthy and fatigued to exercise. If this is the case, we recommend restoring your body's health through correct foods and quality sleep before even starting an exercise program.

18

Enjoy Good Food!

Some of Dr. Berg's Favorite Recipes

Spaghetti Squash with Tahini

Ingredients

- 1 medium spaghetti squash
- ⅓ cup chicken stock
- 4 Tbsp tahini
- 1 tsp finely minced garlic
- 1 Tbsp lemon juice
- 2 Tbsp chopped chives
- Sea salt

Directions

1. Roast the squash at 350 degrees F until the shell can be pierced easily with a fork.

2. Cut the squash in half lengthwise and scoop out seeds. With a fork, gently scrape out the flesh in strands to resemble spaghetti. Keep squash warm.

3. Bring stock to a simmer and stir in tahini, garlic and lemon juice. Toss the squash with the tahini mixture and chives, and salt to taste.

Important note: With all of the recipes, where not specified, it is recommended to use ingredients that are organic/non-GMO and, as applicable, grass-fed or pasture-raised, and sugar-free.

Sugar Snap Peas with Lemon Mustard Dressing

Ingredients

- 1 lb sugar snap peas, cut diagonally into ¼-inch slices
- Juice from 1 medium lemon
- 1 Tbsp Dijon-style mustard
- 6 drops clear stevia
- 5 Tbsp olive oil
- ¼ cup Canadian bacon (unprocessed and organic), julienned
- 2 Tbsp green onions, finely minced
- Sea salt

Directions

1. Bring a pot of salted water to a boil. Add the peas to the boiling water and cook until almost tender but still a little crisp, approx. 3 minutes. Plunge the peas into a bowl of ice water to stop them from cooking further, and drain.

2. Whisk together the lemon juice, mustard, stevia and olive oil; add salt to taste.

3. In a large bowl, gently toss together the peas, Canadian bacon, green onions and dressing.

4. Serve at room temperature.

Asparagus and Tomato Frittata

Ingredients

- 2 eggs
- 1 Tbsp butter
- ½ cup asparagus, sliced diagonally into 1-inch pieces
- 1 medium plum tomato, diced (approx. ½ cup)
- Sea salt

Directions

1. Preheat broiler.
2. Beat eggs in a small bowl with salt.
3. Preheat 8-inch frying pan over medium heat. When pan is hot but not smoking, melt butter.
4. Cook asparagus until just tender, approx. 3 minutes.
5. Add eggs and tomato to the pan and stir with a fork until just blended; add salt to taste.
6. Allow eggs to set on the bottom for 1 to 1½ minutes.
7. Remove the pan from heat and slip under the broiler until the top of the frittata is just set and puffy. Watch closely; this will only take about a minute.
8. Serve immediately.

Sesame Ginger Kale Slaw

Dressing

Ingredients

- ⅓ cup rice vinegar
- 2 Tbsp soy sauce (organic)
- 1 Tbsp Dijon mustard
- 1 Tbsp chopped garlic
- 2 Tbsp minced or grated ginger
- Sea salt
- ¼ cup sesame oil
- ¼ cup safflower oil
- 2 Tbsp sesame seeds

Directions

1. In a blender, combine rice vinegar, soy sauce, mustard, garlic, ginger, and salt to taste. While blender is running, drizzle in the oils and blend well. Stir in sesame seeds. Refrigerate until chilled.

2. Lightly dress shredded or finely chopped kale, shredded carrots, thinly sliced red onion and chopped walnuts (if desired). Toss well before serving.

Kale Slaw

Dressing

Ingredients

- 1 egg
- 2 tsp celery seed
- 1 tsp dry mustard

- ½ tsp sea salt
- ½ cup cider vinegar
- 1½ cups safflower oil

Directions

1. In a blender, combine all ingredients except oil. While blending on high speed, slowly drizzle in the oil. Refrigerate.

2. Just before serving, lightly dress shredded or finely chopped kale, shredded carrots and thinly sliced red onion. Toss well and serve.

Curried Chicken Salad

Ingredients

- 4 cups poached chicken, cut in chunks
- 3 cups sliced celery
- ½ tsp sea salt
- ½ cup sliced almonds
- 2 Tbsp lemon juice
- Curry mayo (see recipe on next page)

Directions

Combine all ingredients. Chill.

Curry Mayonnaise

Ingredients

- 1 large egg
- 1 Tbsp good curry powder
- ½ tsp sea salt
- ¼ tsp freshly ground white pepper
- 1 Tbsp lemon juice
- 1 cup safflower oil

Directions

1. Place everything but the oil in a blender or food processor container. Process 5 seconds in the blender, 15 seconds in the processor.

2. With the motor running, add the oil, first in a drizzle, then in a thin, steady stream. When all the oil has been added, stop the motor and test for consistency. If the sauce is too thick, thin with a small amount of hot water or lemon juice. If too thin, process a little longer.

Walnut Chicken

Ingredients

- 1½ cups walnuts
- 5 cloves garlic, roughly chopped
- ¾ cup boiling water
- 2 tsp red wine vinegar
- ½ tsp sea salt
- 1 tsp crumbled saffron threads
- ¾ tsp ground coriander
- ¼ tsp paprika (preferably Hungarian)
- Dash cayenne pepper
- 6 boneless chicken breasts
- 1–2 Tbsp butter or olive oil

Directions

1. For the sauce: Early in the day, pulse the nuts coarsely in a food processor. Add the garlic and continue to pulse until the mixture is a paste. Transfer to a bowl and gradually stir in the boiling water, stirring constantly until smooth. Stir in the vinegar and spices. Allow to stand several hours for the flavors to blend. Do not refrigerate.

2. When ready to cook chicken, preheat oven to 450 degrees F. Rub chicken breasts with a little butter or olive oil and place in a single layer in a shallow pan.

3. Roast for 20 to 25 minutes till there is no pink remaining.

4. Remove from oven and cover loosely with foil. Allow to rest 10 minutes before slicing. Spoon the sauce over the sliced chicken and serve.

Garlic Walnut Chicken

Ingredients

- 4 bone-in chicken breast halves
- Sea salt
- Freshly ground black pepper
- 2 Tbsp butter
- 1 Tbsp safflower oil
- 10–12 cloves garlic, peeled
- 1 cup walnuts
- 1 cup water

Directions

1. Season the chicken with salt and pepper.
2. In a large skillet, heat the butter and oil. Sauté chicken on each side over medium heat for 3 to 4 minutes. Cover the pan and continue to cook until the chicken is done.
3. Meanwhile, in the food processor, grind the walnuts and garlic until fine, but not a paste.
4. When chicken is done, remove from pan and keep warm.
5. Drain the pan, reserving 4 Tbsp of the drippings. Add the ground garlic and nuts to the pan and sauté on medium heat for 2 minutes. Add the water and simmer for 5 more minutes.
6. Return the chicken to the pan, turning it to coat with the sauce. Heat through before serving.

Chicken with Asparagus

Ingredients

- 4 boneless chicken breast halves
- 1 tsp ground coriander
- Sea salt and freshly ground pepper
- 2 Tbsp olive oil
- 20 asparagus spears
- 1 cup chicken stock
- 1 Tbsp lemon juice
- 1 Tbsp cold butter
- 1 Tbsp chopped parsley

Directions

1. Slice chicken into ¼-inch strips. Sprinkle the chicken strips with salt, pepper and coriander. Heat the oil in a heavy skillet and sauté the chicken in batches for 3 to 4 minutes until lightly browned and all the chicken is cooked. Keep chicken warm.

2. Add the stock and asparagus to the pan and simmer 4 to 5 minutes until the asparagus is nearly tender. Remove from pan and keep warm with chicken.

3. Add lemon juice to juices in pan and swirl in butter to thicken. Pour over chicken and asparagus and sprinkle with parsley.

Chicken Paprikash

Ingredients

- 4 boneless chicken breasts cut in large pieces
- 1 medium onion, finely chopped
- 2 Tbsp safflower oil
- 1 tsp Hungarian paprika
- 1 yellow pepper, halved and sliced
- 1 tomato, halved and sliced
- Sea salt
- 2 Tbsp chopped parsley (optional)

Directions

1. Sauté the onion in oil over medium heat until golden.

2. Remove from heat and sprinkle with paprika. Stir in chicken, yellow pepper, tomato, and salt to taste. Cover and cook gently over medium-low heat until chicken is just done.

3. Remove from heat and serve with a sprinkle of parsley.

Warm Chicken Salad

Ingredients

- 4 boneless chicken breasts
- ½ lb snow peas
- 6 cups mixed lettuce, washed and dried
- 3 carrots, peeled and cut into julienne pieces
- 2 cups sliced button mushrooms
- 1 Tbsp chopped cilantro

Dressing/Marinade

- ½ cup lemon juice
- 2 Tbsp whole-grain mustard
- 1 cup olive oil
- 4 Tbsp sesame oil
- 1 tsp ground coriander

Directions

1. Mix all dressing ingredients together.
2. Place chicken in a shallow container with half the dressing. Cover tightly and refrigerate 8 hours or overnight.
3. Store the remaining dressing in the refrigerator.
4. Broil the chicken until cooked through. Allow to rest 10 minutes.
5. Cook the snow peas in boiling water for 2 minutes, drain and run under cold water to stop cooking process.

Assembling the Salad

- Tear the lettuce into bite-sized pieces and combine with the other vegetables in a serving bowl.
- Slice the chicken thinly and distribute over the salad. Toss with dressing and sprinkle with chopped cilantro.

Chicken with Herbed Cheese

Ingredients

- 4 boneless chicken breast halves
- ½ cup ricotta cheese
- 1 egg, beaten
- 2 Tbsp minced parsley and chives or other herbs as desired
- 1 tsp crushed garlic
- 1 tsp minced onion
- Sea salt
- Freshly ground pepper
- 3 Tbsp melted butter

Directions

1. Preheat oven to 450 degrees F.
2. With a sharp knife, cut a pocket in each chicken breast.
3. In a small bowl, combine the cheese with the egg and mix thoroughly. Stir in the herbs, garlic and onion.
4. Using a small spoon, stuff each breast with several tablespoons of the cheese mixture. Fasten with toothpicks if necessary. Season both sides with salt and pepper and arrange in a single layer in an oiled shallow roasting pan. Pour melted butter over the breasts.
5. Bake for approximately 25 minutes or until chicken is no longer pink. Turn once when halfway done to brown both sides. Let chicken rest 5 minutes before serving.

Easy Meatloaf

Ingredients

- 2 lbs extra-lean ground beef
- 6–8 oz portobello mushroom caps
- 2 eggs
- ½ cup medium hot salsa*
- 1½ tsp sea salt
- 1 tsp pepper

Directions

1. Preheat oven to 375 degrees F.
2. Mince mushroom caps in a food processor until very fine.
3. In a large bowl, stir together minced mushrooms, eggs, salsa, salt and pepper.
4. If salsa is chunky, break up large pieces.
5. Using your hands, thoroughly mix ground beef with mushroom mixture.
6. In a shallow baking dish, form meat mixture into a loaf. Bake for one hour or until internal temperature reaches 160 degrees F.

---

* Picante sauce or *pico de gallo* can be substituted.

Healthy Pleasure Foods

Legal Brownies

Amazing brownies that
have no flour or sugar

Ingredients

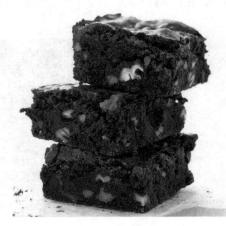

- 2 sticks butter or 1 stick butter
  and ½ cup coconut butter
- ½ cup cocoa powder
  (unsweetened)
- 1 cup chopped walnuts
- ⅔ cup or ¾ cup xylitol
  sweetener (depending on
  how sweet you like it)

- 4 eggs (whole)
- 1 tsp vanilla extract

Directions

1. Preheat oven to 375 degrees F.
2. Melt the butter (or coconut butter).
3. On low speed, mix butter, cocoa powder, walnuts, xylitol, eggs and
   vanilla until batter is smooth and fluffy; this can take a few minutes.
4. Grease a glass or metal 8″ x 8″ square pan with butter or coconut butter.
5. Pour mixture evenly into the baking pan.
6. Bake for 20 to 25 minutes and put toothpick in center to see if
   brownie mix sticks. If the toothpick comes out clean, the brownies
   are fully cooked.
7. Remove and let cool for 15 minutes.
8. These brownies must be kept in the refrigerator because they contain
   butter, which tends to melt at room temperature.

Cauliflower Hot Wings

If you like hot wings, you'll love these!

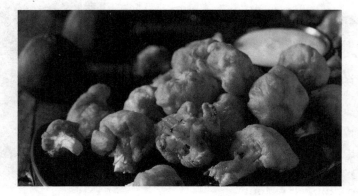

Ingredients

- 1 head / 2 to 3 lbs / 8 to 12 cups cauliflower
- 1 cup / 8 oz organic milk
- ¾ cup / 3 oz almond flour

- 2 tsp garlic powder
- 1 Tbsp / ½ oz butter
- 1 cup / 8 oz Frank's RedHot sauce

Directions

1. Preheat oven to 425 degrees F.
2. Cut the cauliflower into bite-sized pieces.
3. In a shallow bowl, stir together milk, almond flour and garlic powder.
4. Dip each piece of cauliflower in the batter and allow the extra batter to drip off.
5. Place on a greased baking sheet.
6. Bake for 20 minutes.
7. Melt the butter in a saucepan over low heat.
8. Mix together the melted butter and Frank's RedHot sauce.
9. Toss cooked cauliflower pieces with the butter and sauce.
10. Serve with a side of blue cheese or ranch dressing.

Cauliflower Mashed

This is your new alternative to mashed potatoes!

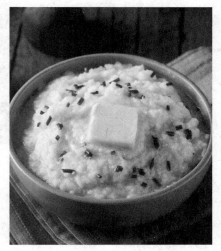

Ingredients

- 1 head / 2 to 3 lb / 8 to 12 cups cauliflower
- 2 oz / 4 tsp / ½ stick butter
- ½ tsp sea salt
- ½ tsp pepper
- ¼ cup chopped chives
- *Optional:* ½ cup / 2 oz organic sharp cheddar cheese

Directions

1. Use only the florets. Cut the stems off the florets of the cauliflower.
2. Bring water to a boil and add the florets.
3. Cook for 20 minutes over medium heat.
4. Mash the cooked cauliflower with the butter, salt and pepper (and cheese if you choose).
5. Serve with a sprinkle of chives and enjoy!

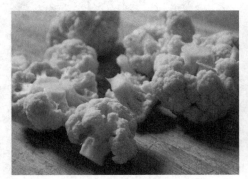
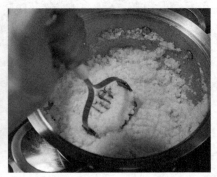

Cauliflower Rice

A rice alternative that is totally healthy

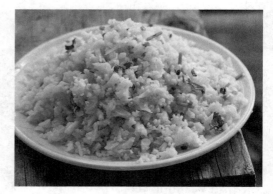

Ingredients

- 1 head / 2 to 3 lb / 8 to 12 cups cauliflower
- ½ cup / 2 oz small onion, chopped
- 1 Tbsp butter
- 1 tsp sea salt
- 1 tsp black pepper
- ¼ cup chopped parsley

Directions

1. Cut the cauliflower into large chunks for grating.
2. Shred the cauliflower with a grater.
3. Chop the onion into small pieces.
4. Sauté the chopped onion in butter until slightly brown.
5. Mix the cauliflower, onion, butter, salt and pepper together.
6. Cook the now-shredded cauliflower mixture in a covered skillet for 10 minutes over low heat until soft.
7. Serve with a sprinkle of parsley and enjoy!

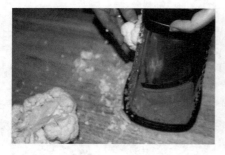
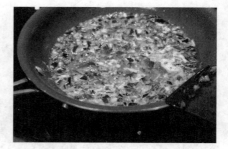

No-Flour Amazing Pizza

Finally, a delicious pizza you can consume, but without the flour crust!

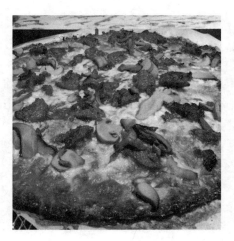

Ingredients

CRUST

- 2 cups / 8 oz grated cauliflower (pregrated weight)
- 2 cups / 8 oz shredded mozzarella cheese (organic)
- 2 eggs
- *Optional:* ½ cup / 2 oz onions, sautéed

TOPPINGS (add what you like)

- ¼ cup / 2 oz pizza sauce or pasta sauce (choose the one with the least amount of sugar)
- 1 cup / 8 oz mozzarella cheese (sprinkle on top)
- Sliced mushrooms (optional)
- Basil leaves (optional) or sausage
- Pepperoni slices (optional)
- Sliced tomatoes (optional)
- Olives (optional)

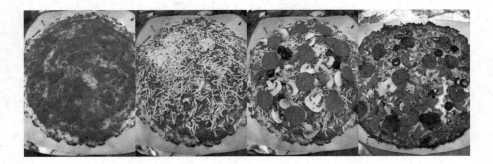

Directions

1. Preheat oven to 450 degrees F.
2. Grate cauliflower.
3. Combine and mix grated cauliflower, eggs and shredded mozzarella cheese in a mixing bowl. This will be the crust of your pizza.
4. Cut parchment paper to fit pizza pan.

Parchment Paper Trick

- To cut a circle of the right size, first tear off a square of parchment roughly the size of the pan. Fold it in half and then fold it in half again.
- Fold the square into a triangle. Find the corner of the triangle where the center of the paper will be once it's unfolded. This is your center point.
- Hold the triangle up to the pan with the center point of the triangle at the middle of the pan.
- Approximate the distance from the middle of the pan to the outer edge and trim off the excess paper, following the curve of the pan.
- Unfold the paper and lay it flat in the pan. Trim any rough edges if it doesn't fit quite right.

5. Mix crust mixture thoroughly and spread on the parchment paper as thinly as possible.
6. Cook the crust for 15 minutes. Let cool down for 5 minutes.
7. Apply sauce, cheese and topping/s.
8. Cook for an additional 10 minutes and enjoy!

Zucchini Pasta

A pasta alternative that will blow you away!

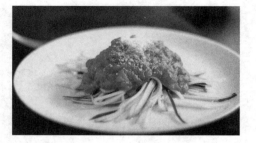

Ingredients

- 2 medium-sized raw zucchini, washed, dried and trimmed at both ends
- 1 cup / 8 oz spaghetti sauce, low-sugar (5 g or less)
- 2 Tbsp / 1 oz freshly squeezed lemon juice
- Parmesan cheese

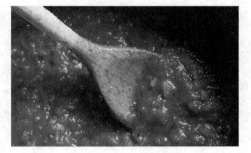

Directions

1. Boil the spaghetti sauce.
2. Shred the zucchini with a peeler.
   - Using a julienne peeler or a spiral vegetable slicer, slice zucchini lengthwise into long, thin strands. Slice the zucchini just until you reach the seeds in the middle and then stop (the seeds will cause the noodles to fall apart). NOTE: If you don't have a julienne peeler or a spiral slicer, you can use a vegetable peeler.
3. Separate the zucchini strands. Transfer zucchini strands to a plate without cooking. Pour lemon juice over zucchini strands.
4. Add spaghetti sauce and sprinkle with Parmesan cheese.

Additional Ideas

- Top with pesto or guacamole.
- Top with grilled shrimp or chicken.

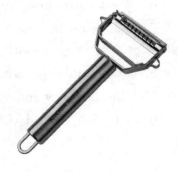

Healthy Pancakes

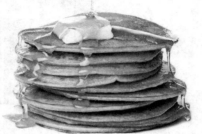

Ingredients

Makes 4 regular or 8 silver-dollar pancakes

- 1 cup almond flour
- 1 Tbsp xylitol sweetener
- ½ tsp baking powder
- ¼ tsp baking soda
- ⅛ tsp sea salt, finely ground

- 1 egg
- 1 Tbsp light olive oil
- ½ cup organic buttermilk
- Softened butter and Joseph's Sugar-Free Maple Syrup, for serving

Directions

1. Preheat a griddle to 375 degrees F.
2. Combine dry ingredients in a large bowl.
3. Lightly whisk egg, then add olive oil and beat well.
4. Add the buttermilk and stir to combine.
5. Add the egg/buttermilk mixture to the dry ingredients and whisk until smooth.
6. Allow batter to sit for at least 2 minutes to rise.
7. Pour 4 medium or 8 small pancakes onto the griddle (silver-dollar size are MUCH easier to flip, especially if you are a novice).
8. Cook until edges are done and bottoms are golden.
9. Turn pancakes and cook about 1 minute longer or until done.
10. Serve hot, topped with butter and sugar-free maple syrup, and enjoy!

Guilt-Free Cookies

Ingredients

- 8 oz (2 sticks) butter (organic, or my favorite: Kerrygold Irish butter)
- 4 Tbsp xylitol sweetener
- 2 cups / 8 oz crushed pecans
- 1 chocolate bar (3.5 oz); must be diabetic chocolate (I like Simply Lite, from Trader Joe's)
- 2 cups / 8 oz almond flour
- 2 tsp vanilla extract
- ¹⁄₁₆ tsp / 1 pinch sea salt

Directions

1. Leave butter out of the refrigerator overnight— must be soft.
2. Preheat the oven to 325 degrees F.
3. Mix the butter with the xylitol by hand until very smooth.
4. Crush the pecans (in grinder, food processor or in a bag with a rolling pin).

   Make sure you have 2 cups of crushed pecans in the final product.

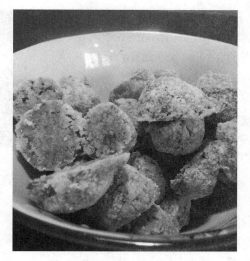

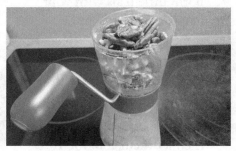

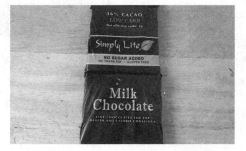

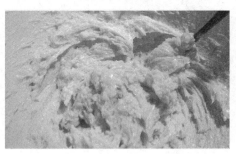

5. Break down (or grind) the chocolate bar in a food processor or by other means.

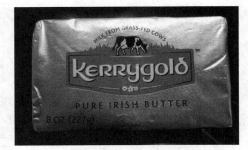

6. Mix thoroughly the sweetened butter, almond flour, crushed pecans, crushed chocolate bar, vanilla extract and sea salt in a bowl. As an option, you could mix it in your food processor.

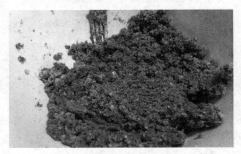

7. Form little balls with your hands and roll them in some almond flour (to coat them), putting them on a cookie sheet lined with parchment paper.

8. Cook for 13 minutes, then let them cool for 10 minutes, then place in the freezer until frozen.

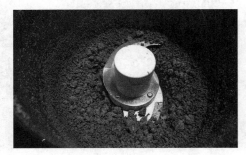

9. Enjoy!!!

Almond Coconut Chocolates

This is a healthy candy
that is totally legal!

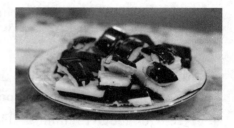

Ingredients

- 1½ cups sugar-free chocolate
  chips (we use Lily's)
- Whole raw almonds
  (can use slivered)
- 4 cups shredded unsweetened
  coconut

- ½ cup to ⅔ cup coconut oil
- Stevia extract (we use
  coconut-flavored)
- Sea salt (optional)

This candy can be made in any order: coconut on the bottom or on
top of the chocolate, nuts inside or on the top. This is totally up to you.
Basically you will prepare one layer, freeze until hard, then the other layer,
and freeze. Below is how I like to do it. But you are the artist in your own
kitchen. Varying it up makes a really pretty display.

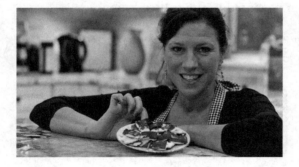

Directions

1. Melt the chocolate chips and 1 tablespoon of coconut oil in a double
   boiler. This will melt fast, so stir often. When completely melted, I
   add about ½ tsp of salt. You don't have to do this, but I *love* a little
   saltiness to my chocolate. If you don't, just leave out the salt.

2. Pour. Once the chocolate is smooth as silk, move over to your molds. Use a spoon and pour a thick layer covering the bottom of your mold. (Be very aware of the depth of your mold and fill no more than one-third deep with chocolate). Do each section of the mold until all the chocolate is used.

3. Almonds are then placed into the chocolate. Don't skimp. The fun is in getting a nice crunch of almonds in every bite!

4. Freeze for about 10 minutes. The candy will be completely hard.

5. Put coconut in a food processor with the coconut oil. Mix until very smooth and almost runny—if too dry, it is harder to work with. Add more coconut oil if necessary. Then add stevia to taste. I add about 7 to 8 drops. It doesn't have to have stevia added, since the chocolate chips are sweet enough. This is really up to your taste. But I do like to add a little sweetness to the coconut. Blend again until all smooth.

6. Pour/spread coconut mixture on top of the frozen chocolate/nuts. Be sure to fill in all areas and cover chocolate.

7. Freeze again until coconut is hard, about 10 minutes.

8. Pop the candy out of the mold, and break the bars into smaller pieces. These can be stored in the fridge. Enjoy!

Candy molds can be purchased at any craft store; we use bars or bud-shaped molds.

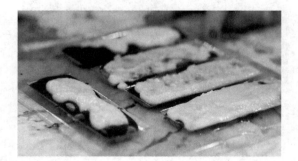

No-Grain English Muffins

These no-grain English muffins are excellent for making sandwiches!

Ingredients

Makes 8 muffins

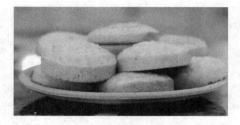

- 1½ cups almond flour
- 6 eggs, beaten
- 6 Tbsp / 3 oz melted butter (grass-fed)
- 1 Tbsp baking powder
- ½ tsp sea salt

Directions

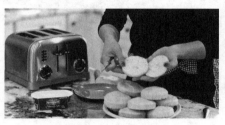

1. Preheat oven to 350 degrees F.

2. In a bowl, stir together all ingredients until thoroughly mixed.

3. Grease muffin rings. Place the rings on a cooking sheet lined with parchment paper or use a silicone baking mat.

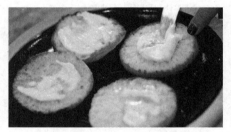

4. Sprinkle a little almond flour on the mat inside each ring. Fill each ring with muffin batter.

5. Bake the muffins for 20 minutes or until they are lightly browned on the top, watching carefully so they do not burn.

6. Allow the muffins to cool for several minutes on the sheet. Once they are firm, use a thin spatula to move the muffins onto a cooling cloth or rack and remove the rings.

7. When ready to serve, fork-split the muffins, butter and lightly brown the inside in a sauté pan. Or toast in a toaster oven and then butter, if desired.

For muffin rings, go to Amazon.com.

Comfort Cookies

These gluten-/flour-free, sugar-free cookies have an amazing texture and flavor. You'll love them!

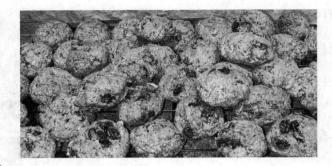

Ingredients

- 2 cups almond meal
- ½ cup flaxseed meal
- ½ cup unsweetened shredded coconut
- ½ cup raw sunflower seeds
- ½ cup raw pumpkin seeds
- 1 Tbsp cinnamon
- 1 tsp sea salt
- 1 tsp baking soda
- 2 eggs (as always, organic, pasture-raised)
- ½ cup Joseph's Sugar-Free Maple Syrup
- 1 tsp vanilla extract
- ½ cup coconut oil, melted

Directions

1. Heat oven to 325 degrees F.
2. In a large bowl, mix all dry ingredients.
3. In another bowl, combine eggs, maple syrup, vanilla and coconut oil. Use a hand mixer to get all the coconut oil really blended.
4. Stir into dry ingredients, and mix.
5. Drop tablespoons of the mixture onto a parchment-lined cookie sheet or a silicone mat. They don't spread, so you can get a lot on one tray.
6. Bake for 15 minutes. Cool on a rack and enjoy.

No-Grain Granola

You'll be asking yourself, "How can something so healthy be so good?"

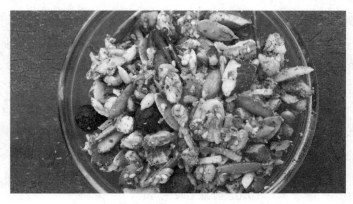

If you think you have a favorite granola recipe, this one will take you by surprise. It's delicious, super filling and EASY to throw together. You can add almond milk and use it as your cereal!

Ingredients

- 2 cups blanched, sliced almonds
- 1 cup pecans
- 1 cup chopped walnuts
- 1 cup sunflower seeds
- 1 cup pepitas (shelled pumpkin seeds)
- ¼ cup sesame seeds
- ¼ cup ground flaxseed or flaxseed meal; you can also use almond meal in place of the flax
- ¾ cup unsweetened coconut flakes
- ½ cup Joseph's Sugar-Free Maple Syrup
- 6 Tbsp coconut oil
- 1 tsp vanilla extract
- 1 tsp cinnamon*
- ½ tsp cloves*
- ½ tsp ground ginger*
- ¹⁄₁₆ tsp / 1 pinch sea salt
- 1 cup organic fresh or dried, unsweetened blueberries

* You can be quite flexible in the choice of spices. We really like this combination, but you could also use nutmeg, allspice, pumpkin pie spice or apple pie spice in amounts to suit your taste.

Directions

1. Preheat oven to 275 degrees F.

2. Lightly grease a sheet pan or, for easy cleanup, line a baking sheet with parchment paper.

3. Combine all the nuts, seeds and coconut in a large bowl.

4. Over low heat, combine sweetener and coconut oil until melted. Remove from heat and stir in vanilla, cinnamon, cloves, ginger and salt.

5. Pour heated ingredients over nut/seed mixture and mix well. Be sure to scrape out all the good sweetener, oil and spices left in the bowl.

6. Spread mixture onto prepared baking sheet.

7. Bake for 45 to 60 minutes or until golden brown, stirring every 15 minutes to keep granola at the edges of the pan from burning. Watch carefully after 45 minutes, as ovens vary.

8. Once the granola is a nice golden brown, remove it from oven and allow it to cool.

9. Add blueberries after granola has cooled.

One last thing: If you like your granola in larger clumps, don't stir it right after it comes out of the oven. Just let it cool on the sheet and then break it apart. If you like it looser, give it a good stir when it comes out of the oven and again after about 10 minutes.

Healthy Peanut Butter Cups

This is a to-die-for twist on the peanut butter cup. It's organic, sugar-free and raw. They are fast to make and STILL take longer to make than they last in the house!

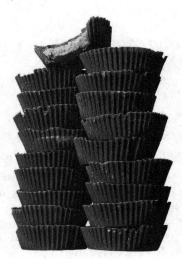

Ingredients

- ¾ cup creamy organic peanut butter
- ½ cup almond flour (more or less)
- Drops of stevia extract
- ¼ tsp sea salt
- 1 cup sugar-free chocolate chips (I use stevia-sweetened)
- 1 Tbsp coconut oil

You'll need a 12-cup muffin tin with paper liners.

Directions

1. Mix the peanut butter and almond flour until smooth and dry enough to make little balls. It can be a bit tacky. If there is too much flour, they will be dry. I like to have them fairly wet and tacky, and I just use two small spoons to work with.

2. Add stevia to taste, along with salt, and mix. The chocolate will be sweet, so I don't add much stevia.

3. Melt the chocolate chips in a double boiler with coconut oil until silky smooth. Stir frequently.

4. Line the muffin tin with paper cups. Fill each paper cup less than halfway with chocolate, using a small spoon.

5. Make a ball of peanut butter mixture and drop into each cup.

6. Pour chocolate on top of each to cover.

7. Freeze for about 20 minutes.

8. Hide them. Enjoy!

Keto Bombs

Ingredients

- 2 sticks grass-fed butter (Kerrygold)
- 1 cup raw organic coconut butter
- *Options:* You can add either 2 scoops of Instant Kale Shake or ¼ cup cocoa powder and ¼ cup xylitol.
- ½ cup Lily's chocolate chips (stevia-sweetened)
- 1 cup pecans (or similar nuts)
- ½ tsp vanilla extract
- ⅛ tsp sea salt

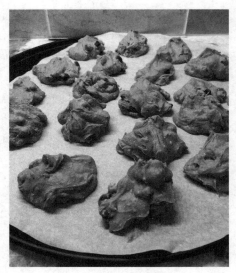

- *Optional:* 1 cup peanut butter/ almond butter (no added sugar)
- *Optional:* 8 oz organic cream cheese

Directions

1. Combine all ingredients and mix thoroughly.
2. Drop teaspoons of the mixture onto a cookie sheet lined with parchment paper and place in the freezer.

These are rich, so you should have only one per day.

No-Sugar Chocolate Ice Cream

Ingredients

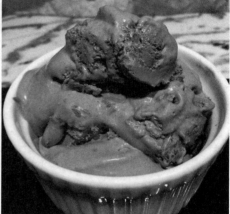

- 2 cups organic heavy cream
- 1 cup coconut milk (organic)
- ½ cup unsweetened
  cocoa powder
- 6 large organic egg yolks
- ⅔ cup sweetener (I recommend
  xylitol or erythritol)
- ⅛ tsp vanilla extract
- ¹⁄₁₆ tsp / 1 pinch sea salt
- ¼ tsp xanthan gum (this helps
  to prevent ice cream from turning into ice in the freezer)
- *Optional:* Chopped pecans (1 cup) and peanut butter (½ cup),
  swirled in

Directions

1. Grind xylitol in a coffee grinder to make into a powder.
2. In a small pot, simmer (not quite at a boil) heavy cream, coconut milk, cocoa powder, sweetener, vanilla, xanthan gum and salt until sweetener completely dissolves, about 5 minutes. Remove pot from heat.
3. In a separate bowl, whisk egg yolks.
4. Whisking constantly, slowly pour about one-third of the hot cream into the yolks, then whisk the yolk mixture back into the pot of cream.
5. Return pot to medium-low heat and gently cook until mixture is thick enough to coat the back of a spoon (about 170 degrees F on an instant-read thermometer).
6. Cool mixture to room temperature. Cover and chill at least 4 hours or overnight, or keep in refrigerator to speed things up.
7. Churn liquid in an ice-cream machine, adding optional ingredients (chopped pecans and peanut butter). Serve directly from the machine for soft serve, or store in freezer until needed.

Low-Carbohydrate Cheesecake

For special occasions. With Liver body types, too many heavy fats will cause bloating—so go light.

Ingredients

- 2 (8-ounce) containers organic cream cheese
- ¼ cup xylitol (non-GMO)
- ⅓ cup organic/grass-fed butter or ⅓ cup melted organic coconut butter
- 2 heaping Tbsp peanut butter (almond butter also works well)
- 1 tsp vanilla extract
- 1⅓ cups ground nut meal (hazelnut, almond or pecan— I like pecan best)
- 2 organic, pasture-raised eggs

Directions

Overview

You will be making a nut crust with cream cheese filler, sweetened with xylitol.

- ○ Set out the two containers of cream cheese, along with the butter or coconut butter, until soft.
- ○ You'll need a pie dish, either glass or enamel.

Making the Crust

The crust can be made from any type of nuts. You could either purchase a nut meal (from Trader Joe's) or crush the nuts yourself. I recommend using pecans, or Bob's Red Mill almond or hazelnut meal. Others (walnuts, cashews) can be used as well.

- ○ To crush them yourself, use a rolling pin and a cutting board. Crush into a meal (small-particle) texture.

1. Into a bowl, add nut meal, butter or coconut butter, and peanut or almond butter.

2. Mix together thoroughly.

3. Place mixture into the pie dish. You do not have to grease the dish, due to the oils.

4. You need to form the crust with your fingers.

Filler

- In a second bowl, add cream cheese, xylitol, vanilla and eggs. Mix together either in a blender or by hand with a fork until creamy.

- An additional step, which is quite good, is to sprinkle some shredded raw organic coconut over the crust, then pour the mixture onto the crust.

5. Preheat oven to 350 degrees F and bake for 30 to 40 minutes.

6. A small crack should appear in the top of the cheesecake, and the top should also begin to turn a slight yellow or light brown. To assess if cooked, you could stick a fork into the center; if no residue clings to the fork, it's done.

7. Let set for 10 minutes to cool.

8. Eat away!

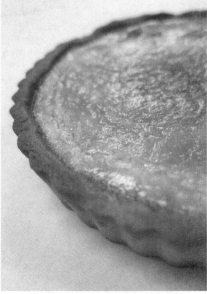

Milkshake Alternative

Dr. Berg's Meal Replacement is made from pea protein and coconut oil powder and sweetened with acceptable, extremely low-glycemic sweeteners (xylitol, erythritol and stevia). Just add water or cold almond milk, shake and drink!

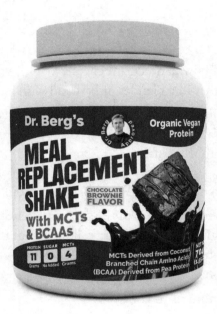

Soda Alternatives

Add 1 dropperful (only 10 drops) of flavored stevia to an 8-ounce bottle of carbonated water (or San Pellegrino or Perrier). It will taste almost like soda, but it's healthy.

My favorite stevia flavors are root beer, cola and lemon, though many flavors are available.

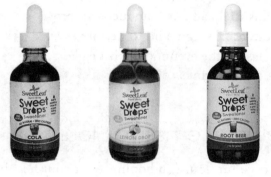

FLAVORED STEVIA

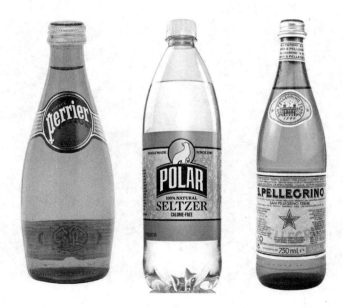

Alcohol, Wine and Beer Alternative

Kombucha tea

Kombucha tea is a great alternative to alcohol because the texture and carbonation mimic beer and wine. It even creates calmness and will help you wind down; plus the acids in kombucha improve your absorption of calcium and other minerals. Drink ½ to 1 glass in the evening in a wine glass.

http://www.synergydrinks.com/

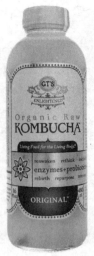

Acceptable Alternative Flours

Almond or coconut flour (find online or at your health food store).

Chocolate Alternatives

If you love chocolate, look for brands sweetened with alternative sweeteners. The sweeteners stevia, xylitol and erythritol are the best.

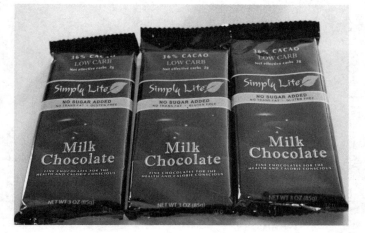

Acceptable Sweeteners

Xylitol, erythritol or stevia (order online at Amazon.com or find them at your health food store).

Joseph's Sugar-Free Maple Syrup is also acceptable (check Amazon.com).

For a liquid sweetener, I use isomalto-oligosaccharides (IMO), a prebiotic fiber (check Amazon.com).

Questions and Answers

How much weight loss is possible per week?

There are two types of weight problems: (1) water and (2) fat. The maximum fat that can be burned per week is between one and two pounds. That's it. The maximum water loss is unlimited. This would explain how some people can lose and gain several pounds within days. Anyone can do any diet and lose water weight, but the true test is how much real fat they can lose. This program is designed to directly achieve that. It also emphasizes sodium and potassium food ratios. If you're only losing one to two pounds per week, it might not be a bad thing; it might actually be normal. And it's important to understand this so you don't get discouraged. Better indicators for improvement would be energy level, sleep quality, digestion and cravings, as these tell if the body is healing.

How do I know if I have water weight or fat?

There is a test called Body Composition, which allows a practitioner to measure body fat versus fluids. Generally, if you weigh a lot and get your body fat tested and it comes out low or normal, then you probably have more fluid weight. A fairly large percentage of male patients at my clinic have more water weight than body fat. Exercise rarely fixes this water problem—diet is the only way. Vegetables are high in potassium, which will allow the fluid to come out gradually over a few months. If you notice a very slow, gradual weight reduction, then you know it is fat, not fluid.

What if I do not lose weight?

If a person has major problems with stress, proteins in the muscles (thighs and buttocks) can be broken down and turned into sugar. Sugar is then turned into fat around the abdomen. Some people actually gain weight before they lose weight because the body has to rebuild muscle first, and muscle is heavier than fat. Some of our patients lose inches, increase energy and have better digestion, yet they see no initial weight loss. After these muscles are repaired, I have found that weight loss is easier. Nevertheless, it cannot occur until the body is out of stress mode and in healing mode, and for some people actual weight loss will be delayed for as much as four to eight weeks.

What if I'm pregnant? Can I do this program?

Yes; stick to the basic eating plan in chapter 11. Make sure you are taking some sea kelp and trace minerals if you are pregnant. These are the nutrients that are essential in creating a healthy body. What you eat when you are pregnant will determine the baby's health later.

Can I come off my hormone therapy and medications when I'm on this program?

That is between you and your doctor. As you improve, get him or her to help you make the transition.

What if I'm on medication (e.g., Coumadin) that conflicts with consuming certain vegetables?

The medication Coumadin acts like a vitamin K blocker, preventing the clotting of blood. It's used as a blood thinner to prevent clots and strokes. It is also used as a rat poison. Check with your doctor as to what vegetables you can or cannot eat on this program.

Do I have to avoid taking my supplements on this program?

I would recommend that you only avoid them if they are synthetics. Replace them with whole-food-based vitamins.

What vitamins should I take?

I always recommend a food-based vitamin. Look on the back of the label to see if it mentions actual food; then look at the individual ingredients and notice the milligram amounts. If the vitamins are synthetic, you will see the same number of milligrams for each vitamin; for example: 100 milligrams of B_1, 100 milligrams of B_2, 100 milligrams of B_6. The whole-food vitamins come in different amounts; for instance: 21 milligrams of B_1, 3.4 milligrams of B_2, or 13 milligrams of B_6.

Your program seems very strict. I'm not sure if I can do it.

Something is better than nothing. Do what you can and try to improve your eating each week, making gradual improvements over time. Many people find that the program becomes easier as they see more and more results. Also, as your cravings diminish and you feel more energy, it will be easier to do. Something is better than nothing.

Do I need to buy all organic, hormone-free foods?

I'm not saying you need to change your entire diet overnight; I'll give you a week. Just kidding. It would be ideal to eat only organic, but 50 percent would be the bare minimum. The first change in your diet needs to be consuming hormone-free foods. Then once this is implemented, start adding the organic (non-insecticide) foods.

I can't afford the organic foods. What should I do?

Get a part-time job to support your new diet. I'm kidding again. You could start with just purchasing organic meats, even hamburger and eggs, and keep everything else commercial. The point? The cost is an investment and it will pay off later. You are basically creating a higher level of health, and it's worth the investment. Instead of getting that oil change for your car, buy some organic salad.

The overall protein amounts seem extremely low. Isn't it recommended that a person consume 9 grams per 20 pounds of weight?

Because the cause of stubborn weight is a failing endocrine system, I have found that people can process (digest) less protein than they might have considered. I'm not concerned necessarily about the excess protein adding calories. My concern is that overweight people have poor livers, and too much protein stresses the liver. What benefit is there in adding protein if they are not digesting it? It becomes more of a toxin than a healing food. They actually need more raw whole vegetables. I want them to get their calories from eating lots of vegetables, because it is these vegetables that provide the healing building blocks to repair gland tissue.

What if I get constipated?

This is usually because you're digestive microbes are not used to all this fiber. Microbes live on fiber, and adding in new types of vegetables like kale and so forth can overwhelm the system and back it up. Switch to vegetables that you know you are used to and very gradually add more of the new.

What do I do if I'm allergic to the foods recommended?

Occasionally, a person might think he or she is allergic or has sensitivity to some of the foods recommended, such as broccoli and cabbage. This is more a missing enzyme than an allergy. The person lacks the enzyme needed to digest certain foods, adding stress and bloating to the system and causing gas in the intestines. I believe this is the result of eating too many cooked and pasteurized foods, which over the years deplete your enzyme reserves. That is why it is important to germinate (soak in water overnight) your seeds and nuts to remove enzyme inhibitors, so that the enzymes in the foods can be reactivated, causing less dependency on your own enzyme reserves.

Common gas-producing foods are beans, artichokes, asparagus, broccoli, Brussels sprouts, cabbage, cauliflower, cucumbers, green peppers, onions, radishes, bananas, apricots and pears. Consume vegetables you know do not cause bloating, as this intestinal stress can increase stress hormones, preventing weight loss.

Make a food log to track your responses and start replacing foods that you are sensitive to with foods you know you can eat without the bloating. Many people are sensitive to cashew nuts, which make them feel bloated and tired. I think this is because most cashews one buys are cooked or roasted, which puts more strain on the body's enzyme reserves. If you experience bloating with any foods, either germinate them (if nuts or seeds) or avoid them, or you can add the missing enzyme to digest these foods—go to http://www.bean-zyme.com/.

What if I just don't like vegetables or can't get enough in my diet?

It is highly recommended that you consume as many vegetables as you can. However, there is something you could do to make up for the lack of quantity. You could consume better-quality nutrition, like sprouts. A small serving of sprouts gives you just as much nutrition as a larger quantity of mature vegetables. So you wouldn't be eating as much, just a better quality to get the same nutrition. Eat a small bowl of sprouts with salad dressing.

I'm not hungry for breakfast. Is it okay to skip it?

Absolutely. You do not want to eat if you're not hungry. Your body is already eating its own fat, so you are using your reserves. Only eat when you are hungry.

I thought eggs were bad for me and would give me high cholesterol.

Eggs will not increase cholesterol because they are loaded with the antidote—lecithin. I've been eating eggs for the past 27 years without any problem whatsoever, and my cholesterol levels have stayed below 200.

Your body actually makes 3,000 milligrams of cholesterol every day. That is equal to 333 strips of bacon, or a pound of butter or 14 eggs. When you eat foods high in cholesterol, your body makes less. When you eat less, your body makes more.

Should I consume just the egg white and skip the yolk?

Eat the whole thing. You need this cholesterol to help with building hormones, especially the adrenal hormones. And the more stress you go through, the more fatty foods, especially eggs, I would recommend. Cholesterol also helps in supporting normal nerve and brain function.

Can I eat eggs daily without a problem?

Yes.

What do I do if I get fatigued on this plan?

It means that you either need vitamin B5 or need to switch up your vegetables. Too much kale can make people tired if they can't digest it and get bloated.

What can I do for itching around different parts of my body, including the soles of my feet?

Itching can be a sign of liver issues. When the liver can no longer break down histamines, you experience itching. I recommend taking two amino acids—one called glycine and the other, taurine. These both improve liver function.

Why don't you consider calories within this program?

Calories, which are the units of energy in foods, are rather insignificant, in my opinion, compared to the hormone influence of foods and activities. Let's take fat. Fat has high calories compared to other foods, but fat does *not* stimulate fat-storing hormones. However, carbohydrates like breads or pasta can trigger fat-storing hormones. Cutting calories *can* cause long-term weight gain by stimulating the stress hormone cortisol, which releases sugar in the blood and triggers insulin to change this sugar into fat. That is why some people who go on low-calorie diets gain weight down the road.

You don't seem to put emphasis on the dangers of fats. Why?

Hydrogenated fats are bad, no doubt. But both fat-storing and fat-burning hormones treat fats as neutral, despite their having the most calories.

Is there a way to speed up getting rid of cellulite-type fat on my thighs?

This is usually an Ovary body shape. It can be one of two problems: (1) excessive estrogen or (2) fluid retention within the lymphatic system in the outer thighs. If your eyes are puffy and feel swollen, suspect lymphatic fluid retention. If you press around your bellybutton, you can usually feel some soreness due to congested lymph nodes.

The high potassium in vegetables (7–10 cups) will balance the sodium. The key is to avoid artificial sweeteners and food chemicals and go as natural as possible.

Fibroids and ovarian cysts can produce excess estrogen; so can HRT and birth-control pills. Growth hormones in animal meats can also contain estrogen. Make sure everything is organic and without hormones.

Another tip for this problem is to increase circulation by exercising the lower part of the body as opposed to the top part. Increasing protein in the diet can also decrease water retention.

I'm gaining weight on this diet. What does that mean?

Chances are you are not digesting the large quantities of vegetables on this plan. Reduce and change them to vegetables you know you can digest.

I don't have time to exercise. Can I still lose weight on this program?

Yes, but the six fat-burning hormones have triggers; and the more you can trigger these hormones, the more weight you will lose. If you don't exercise, then you have to keep the diet really perfect. If the diet is not great, then you need to exercise more. If you're not sleeping well, then your diet and exercise need to be even better to compensate for this.

What's the best way to speed up my metabolism with exercise?

Once you graduate from the aerobic light-resistance-type exercise, you can really pick up the pace on anaerobic exercise. The key is to know that *intensity* is the most important trigger. The more intense the exercise, the more the hormone release. Do short, quick intense exercises with lots of rest in between.

I can't sleep at night. Any recommendations?

See the Resources section for recommendations. Also, eat four stalks of celery before bed. Celery contains active compounds called pthalides, which relax the muscles of the arteries that regulate blood pressure. Pthalides also reduce adrenal (stress) hormones, which cause high blood pressure. When researchers injected a compound derived from celery into test animals, the animals' blood pressure dropped 12–14 percent. In humans, an equivalent dose would be supplied by about four stalks of celery.*

You could also try kombucha tea, which is a friendly bacteria and yeast product, obtainable at a health food store in the refrigerated section. It balances your pH and greatly helps sleeping. However, certain people start craving more sweet foods when they drink it, while others don't; so you'll have to judge for yourself.

---

* *Source:* George Mateljan Foundation, *The World's Healthiest Foods:* Celery.

Do I burn more fat when I sleep?

Fat is released via hormones, especially growth hormone. Growth hormone is active during the night while you sleep, but to get the most benefit from its fat-burning effects you should go to bed before 11:00 p.m.

Why do pain and lack of sleep keep me from weight loss?

Pain and lack of sleep trigger cortisol, which keeps you out of fat burning. If pain or stress is keeping you from sleeping, I would recommend going to my YouTube channel and searching for those problems, and you'll most likely find a video on this.

How much water should I drink per day?

Don't ever force yourself to drink water. Drink when you are thirsty.

Is it true that consuming beef will cause cancer?

From the research I have done, a prime cause of cancer is low oxygen in the cells, which leads to alteration in the DNA and then cancer. Certain fats, called omega fatty acids, make up our cellular membranes, especially the parts that control cell respiration (breathing of oxygen). If you starve the cells of the raw materials they need in order to breathe, it seems obvious that your risk for cancer can increase. Commercial beef (grain-fed) has very low levels of omega-3 fatty acids, which are protective to your cell walls. However, when you consume grass-fed beef, omega-3 fats are much higher and hence cancer protective.

Is there a difference between farm-raised fish and wild-caught fish?

Big time! Each category has both omega-3 and omega-6 fats, which need to be in a certain ratio, but wild-caught fish have far more omega-3 fatty acids, in addition to being free of the hormones fed to farm-raised fish. So, if possible, consume wild-caught fish.

What are the benefits of broccoli sprouts?

Researchers estimate that broccoli sprouts contain *10 to 100 times the power of mature broccoli* to boost enzymes that detoxify potential carcinogens! So a healthy serving of broccoli sprouts in your salad or sandwich can offer even more protection against cancer than larger amounts of full-grown broccoli.

Broccoli sprouts are more nutritious than alfalfa sprouts. However, all sprouts contain much higher levels of nutrition than seeds and grown plants. For example, vitamin C is close to zero in seeds, whereas sprouting releases a huge amount of vitamin C.

Can I overdo eating nuts?

Yes. This is one of the most common problems, as many people stuff their bodies with nuts all day long and then feel bloated, especially when they're falling asleep. Roasted nuts and cashews usually cause the biggest problem; it's difficult to overdo walnuts or almonds. And people generally do better on raw nuts than on roasted nuts and peanut butter.

Heaviness in the abdomen, bloating or gas as a result of eating nuts is caused by the enzyme inhibitors they inherently contain. The way to handle this is to soak the nuts overnight in water to activate these enzymes and start the process of germination. (Details on how to do this are given in chapter 11.) Germinating nuts before you eat them will not only take the stress off your digestive system; it will also provide you with maximum nutrition.

Can I use spices?

Yes, but make sure they don't contain MSG. It comes in other forms: modified food starch, hydrolyzed protein, hydrolyzed vegetable protein, carrageenan, glutamic acid, autolyzed yeast and natural flavorings.

Avoid table salt and use sea salt.

I thought salt was bad for me; why do you recommend it for Adrenal body types?

With adrenal weakness you lose salt, so you need to replace it. Again, use sea salt, not table salt.

What do I do if I'm craving salty foods?

Add some sea salt to your diet every day until the cravings go away. This is usually indicative of adrenal weakness. Sometimes these same cases also crave licorice.

What can I have as a sugar substitute?

The goal is to avoid all sugars, but now and then you have a birthday or other occasion where you are forced to eat some. If this occurs, the following are the best choices, listed in descending order:
- Stevia
- Xylitol (non-GMO)
- Erythritol (non-GMO)

What about the sugar in salad dressing, gum, ketchup, etc.?

You need to start reading labels and look at the sugar amounts. It's these hidden sugars that add up to no weight loss. I get all my condiments at the health food store. Even many brands of pickles have sugar added—so read labels.

What about popcorn?

Popcorn is starch, although it has fiber; but it's best to cut it out completely.

If you're addicted, you can have some every blue moon; however, make sure you add real butter to slow the insulin response. If you find you are not losing weight, then cut it out altogether.

What about puffed cereals or puffed rice cakes?

A few years ago I did an experiment on mice, using four different types of food. Each of the four groups of mice was fed either mouse food, whole-wheat bread, white bread or puffed cereal. Take a wild guess which group died first?

The puffed-cereal group died first, and then the whole-wheat group died next. Paul A. Stitt, author of *Beating the Food Giants*, mentioned that a chemical is released when the cereal is puffed, making it toxic to mice.

Avoid anything puffed.

Can't I eat whole-wheat bread?

Commercial whole-wheat bread has more chemicals and bug sprays (insecticides) than white bread because it has more nutrition for the bugs to live on. It's too much starch and it will slow your progress.

Will I ever be able to eat bread?

Once you achieve your ideal weight and size, you can add occasional bread into your diet. The kind of bread will be Ezekiel or spelt bread, as it is the least damaging to your system. Some other diet programs have several phases that gradually add the processed and refined foods back into the diet. The goal with our program is to get your body used to eating healthful foods, and then maintain that healthy eating.

Another problem with commercial bread is that not only is it too much of a starch but it is also badly processed. The flour most breads are made from loses its vitamins very soon after the grain is ground. Then synthetic vitamins are sprayed onto it. When you eat it, a depletion of these vitamins can occur. Once you achieve your ideal weight you could, in your spare time, grind some wheat fresh and make your own bread—a limited amount.

What about milk or dairy products?

Small amounts are all right to eat if the milk is organic. Cheese and cottage cheese are okay. However, consume organic cottage cheese because commercial cottage cheese contains modified food starch (MSG). Cheese higher in fat, like Brie, is recommend more than low-fat cheese. But yogurt has 6 to 10 grams of sugar per serving size, even in the "plain" flavor. Occasionally you can consume kefir, which has more health benefits than yogurt.

What about consuming soy products?

Most soy in America is genetically modified. It's in almost every product. Soy is badly processed and can increase estrogen. Occasional miso soup is okay. I heard of a man who ate so much soy he started lactating (releasing breast milk).

What about GMO foods?

Genetically modified foods are becoming a problem in the U.S. I would recommend getting a video called *The Future of Food* by going to www.thefutureoffood.com.

Four of the main foods that are being genetically modified presently are soy, corn, canola and sugar beets. It makes you wonder if this is why so many people have allergies to these foods. Manufacturers are not currently regulated or required to mention if the food is GMO or not, which is scary. The only reason they don't want you to know is because you would not buy it.

I've heard that spinach, kale and other leafy greens produce oxalates, which make kidney stones.

This can occur if the leafy green vegetables—especially spinach—are cooked or processed. When these vegetables are eaten *raw*, the oxalic acid they contain may be beneficial in the cleansing and healing of the intestinal tract; but when they are cooked or processed, heat changes the organic (plant-based) acid into an inorganic acid that is no longer plant-based, which binds readily with calcium and other minerals to form oxalates (salts of oxalic acid). Because oxalates are not nutrients, the blood will transport them directly to the kidneys to excrete as urine. If the urine contains large amounts of calcium oxalate, this can solidify into crystals, which, in turn, contribute to the formation of kidney stones.

However, consuming apple cider vinegar and lemon juice or asparagus will act to counter the production of these stones. The benefits of cruciferous and other leafy green vegetables far outweigh the possibility of developing stones; and if the diet is balanced, as we recommend, and the majority of these vegetables are eaten raw, your risks are greatly lowered. But if you have stones, definitely start including the above drinks and food in your diet.

What about a fruit or vegetable juice cleanse?

No way—all that concentrated juice is far too much sugar. I used to juice every day and my health started going downhill. When you eat fruits or vegetables, eat the whole thing. I will say, though, out of all the juices, carrot is the least damaging; but drinking carrot juice in such a concentrated form still gives you too much sugar.

However, there are some exceptions to juicing. For people who are very sick or have lots of fluid retention, as seen in their ankles, it is recommended that they juice fresh vegetables one to two times per day. These would include a combination of celery, carrot, beet, radish, red potato and some kale. Do not store this juice in the refrigerator; it has to be consumed right away to get the full benefit of the enzymes.

What can I do for caffeine withdrawal?

Realize it will last only one to two days—three days at the most. This can happen with some people, particularly if they come off coffee cold turkey. Just schedule this change when you are home over a weekend so you don't get too irritable with those around you. And if you do get grouchy at someone, don't mention my name.

What about decaffeinated coffee?

It is okay in small amounts if it's water processed and organic. Commercial decaf is filled with chemicals.

What about occasional alcoholic beverages?

Alcohol definitely sets the liver back by several days. The least damaging alcoholic beverage is low-carb light beer. The next is a white wine. Some people have the idea that drinking wine will help give them antioxidants. Yes, it may, but the damage to their livers is a bigger concern. You might also say, "People in Europe consume wine. Why can't I?" In most cases, Europeans have not been damaged by growth hormones. Their bodies are stronger and can handle small amounts of wine. If your hormone system is weak, you don't have this option yet.

How do I keep the weight off, now that I've lost it?

The goal of this program is to stabilize your organs so you can keep the weight off. The problem is not your weight; it's your hormones. This is a lifestyle change, and as you get healthier, going back to junk food won't feel right because your taste buds won't be able to tolerate much sugar.

What is the biggest reason why people gain the weight right back?

They lose weight and don't continue a good eating program long enough to achieve full stabilization of a healthy body.

Acknowledgments

I would like to thank Rosemary Delderfield and Janet Stephens for their excellent work in editing and proofreading this book. They have contributed to the clarity of my message and were always one step ahead of me in completing this project. I would also like to acknowledge Allen Harris, the artist, for a fantastic job of illustrating these concepts, along with my wife, Karen, and Kathleen Frascella for their contributions in the testing and compiling of recipes for the book.

Glossary

acesulfame K. Sold commercially as Sunett or Sweet One, it was approved as a sugar substitute by the FDA in 1988. Acetoacetamide, a breakdown product, has been shown to affect the thyroid of rats, rabbits and dogs. This chemical may increase cancer risk in humans.

Addison's disease. Also called adrenal insufficiency or hypocortisolism, this disease occurs when the adrenal glands do not produce enough of the hormone cortisol and, in some cases, the hormone aldosterone. It is characterized by weight loss, muscle weakness, fatigue, poor immune system, low blood pressure, and sometimes the darkening of both exposed and non-exposed skin.

adipose tissue. Fat tissue whose primary function is that of a fuel reserve or fuel storage and whose secondary function is to insulate and cushion. The brain, glands, hormones, nerves and cell walls are made of adipose tissue.

adrenal(s). The two adrenal glands sit on top of the kidneys. Their external outer portion is called the cortex, and the inner portion is called the medulla. Each area produces its own set of hormones.

adrenaline. Hormone produced by the inner part of the adrenal glands (adrenal medulla). Adrenaline has a wide range of functions. It constricts the blood vessels in some parts of the body and dilates them in others. It is involved in stress responses, maintains blood flow to all parts of the body, relaxes the smaller branches of the bronchial tubes, improving oxygen exchange, and causes shivering to generate body heat. In addition, it releases stored sugar in the body to maintain consistent energy. Also called epinephrine.

aerobic exercise. A slow-paced type of exercise (below 130 heartbeats per minute) designed to promote the supply and use of oxygen by the body. Aerobic exercise is considered endurance-type rather than intense exercise. In the first 20 to 30 minutes, stored sugar is used as fuel; after 30 minutes, fat can be tapped into. *Aerobic* in this context means "with oxygen." It derives from the Greek *aer*, "air," and *bios*, "life," + *-ic*, meaning "produced by" or "caused by."

agave nectar. Natural low-calorie sweetener that comes from the cactus plant. It is a stronger sweetener than sugar yet is absorbed into the bloodstream even more slowly than honey.

amino acids. The building blocks of protein. Twenty amino acids are needed to build the various proteins used in the growth, repair and maintenance of body tissues. Eleven of these, the *non-essential amino acids*, can be manufactured by the body, whereas the other nine—known as *essential amino acids*—must come from food. Amino acids form the raw material for a number of hormones. Some amino acids trigger fat-burning hormones (e.g., growth hormone).

anaerobic exercise. An intense resistance-type exercise that involves a higher pulse rate (greater than 145 heartbeats per minute). During the workout, energy is produced without utilizing oxygen and the only source of fuel is sugar in the blood or stored sugar in the muscles and liver. Fat is not burned while exercising; however, fat-burning hormones are stimulated 14 to 48 hours later. *Anaerobic* means "without oxygen"—from the Greek *an-*, "without," *aer*, "air," and *bios,* "life," + *-ic*, meaning "produced by" or "caused by."

androgens. Hormones produced by several glands (adrenals, testicles and ovaries), which are responsible for the male characteristics. *Andro-* means "man" + *-gen*, "something that produces."

anti-carcinogenic. Fights, prevents or blocks cancer. Cruciferous vegetables have anti-carcinogenic properties.

anti-estrogenic. Inhibits or blocks estrogen. Certain cruciferous vegetables have this effect because they help the liver detoxify estrogen.

anti-inflammatory. "Against inflammation"—suppressing or reducing inflammation. The adrenal glands produce hormones that have anti-inflammatory effects.

ascites. A condition involving accumulation of fluid in the abdominal sac (tissue surrounding abdominal organs). Ascites can be caused by a failing liver, kidney or pancreas.

ascorbic acid. Part of the vitamin C complex known as the antioxidant portion.

aspartame. Artificial sweetener marketed under a number of trademark names, such as NutraSweet and Equal; it is an ingredient in approximately 6,000 consumer foods and beverages sold worldwide. Several thousand reports have been submitted to the FDA by both patients and doctors, complaining of 92 different adverse health effects attributed to aspartame.*

atrophy. Breakdown and shrinkage of an organ, gland or muscle, which can occur as a result of excessive hormone secretion, such as cortisol.

autoimmunity. A condition in which the body produces antibodies that attack its own cells and tissues. Normally, adrenal hormones are supposed to suppress immune cells, but when this function is broken, the immune system can go out of control. Autoimmune diseases result from a hyperactive immune system attacking normal tissues as if they were foreign organisms.

autolyze. To undergo, or cause to undergo, autolysis—the destruction of cells or tissues by an organism's own enzymes, as after a disease or death. Also called *self-digestion*. Autolysis is used as a method of producing yeast extract.

biopsy. The removal of bits of tissue from a living body for examination.

calorie. Derived from the Latin word *calor*, meaning "heat," calorie refers to the amount of energy in a food. Different foods of the same quantity contain higher or lower amounts of energy (calories).

---

* *Source:* U.S. Department of Health & Human Services (1993).

candida. A yeast-like fungus that is normally in balance with other friendly microbes. However, an overgrowth of candida can occur after antibiotic use.

capillary. Any of the tiny blood vessels that connect the smallest arteries with the smallest veins.

carbohydrate. Any of a group of substances made of carbon, hydrogen and oxygen, including the sugars, fibers and starches, used by the body as an energy source. There are several types of carbohydrates: grains, vegetables, fruits and sugars. Unrefined carbohydrates provide vitamins and minerals as well as fiber, while refined grains, in the form of breads, pasta, cereals, crackers, donuts and the like, have little nutrient value.

carcinogen. A substance that causes or is capable of causing cancer. Examples are pesticides, insecticides, herbicides, fungicides, plastics, solvents and heavy metals.

carrageenan. A thickening compound extracted from seaweed and red algae, used in some dairy products to stabilize the color and flavor. It often contains MSG and has been linked to digestive upset.

cartilage. Tough elastic tissue assisting in the support of joints.

caseinate. A chemical made from milk protein (casein) and used to stabilize certain foods.

cholesterol. A substance that occurs in egg yolks, meats and dairy products. It is also made by the liver and many other body cells and is an important raw material in the production of hormones. Cholesterol supplies the material to make nerves, brain tissue and endocrine tissue. It also allows nerve transmission, healing and immune system functions. Seventy-five percent of the cholesterol in the body is made by the liver and cells; only 25 percent comes from outside dietary sources. Excessively low cholesterol can weaken the immune system. LDL (bad cholesterol) is a term used to describe the cholesterol going into the liver. HDL (good cholesterol) is a term describing cholesterol coming out of the liver.

circadian rhythm. A rhythmic cycle in the body that occurs roughly every 24 hours. Linked to the light-dark cycle, circadian rhythms are important in determining the sleeping and feeding patterns of all animals, including human beings. Patterns of brain-wave activity, hormone production, cell regeneration and other biological activities are also connected to this daily cycle. The term *circadian* comes from the Latin *circa*, "about," and *dies*, "day," meaning literally "about a day."

cirrhosis. Chronic condition of the liver in which normal tissue is replaced by fibrous scar tissue and normal function is inhibited.

collagen. The main structural protein found in skin, ligaments, tendons, bone, cartilage and other connective tissue. It is the most abundant protein in mammals, making up about 25 percent of the total protein content. Collagen consists of groups of strong white inelastic fibers, enabling these body structures to withstand forces that stretch them. Since it is responsible for skin strength and elasticity, its deterioration leads to wrinkles that accompany aging. Derived from French *collagène*, from Greek *kola*, "glue," + *-gen*, "something that produces," the word *collagen* means "glue producer" and refers to the early process of boiling the skin and sinews of horses and other animals to obtain glue.

cortisol. Important hormone produced by the adrenal glands to counter stress responses. It is anti-inflammatory and releases glucose from the liver and muscles into the blood to help the body respond to stress. It also suppresses immune cells (white blood cells) and is involved in sleep cycles. Cortisol is an indirect fat-making hormone; when it releases excess glucose into the blood, this causes abnormally high insulin levels to convert the sugar into fat around the abdominal organs.

cruciferous. A group of vegetables belonging to the cabbage family, which includes cabbage, bok choy, collards, broccoli, Brussels sprouts, kohlrabi, kale, mustard greens, turnip greens and cauliflower. These leafy green vegetables contain more phytochemicals (plant chemicals) than any other food, which may strengthen the immune system and thereby help build resistance against viruses and diseases. The term is derived from the Latin word *crux*, meaning "cross," because the four petals of these plants' tiny flowers resemble a cross.

cyst. A sac-like structure in plants and animals. In certain abnormal conditions, this sac becomes filled with fluid or disease matter.

delta-wave sleep. Slow-wave or deep sleep, which occurs mostly in the first third of the night. A delta wave is a large, slow electrical brain wave, marking the deepest level of sleep.

detoxification. The removal of poisons or toxins from the body.

diastolic. Refers to when the heart is in a period of relaxation and dilation (expansion). In a blood pressure reading the diastolic pressure is the second number recorded. For example, if the reading is 120/80, the bottom number is the diastolic measurement. By "80" is meant 80 millimeters of mercury. This number measures the pressure against the blood vessel walls when the heart is between beats and resting. Derived from the Greek *diastol*, "expansion," "dilation," from *dia*, "apart" + *stellein*, "to put." See also **systolic**.

diet. 1. The usual food and drink consumed by a person or animal. **2.** A regulated course of food and drink to promote health or for weight control. The word *diet* comes from the Old French *diète*, from Latin *diaeta*, which means "way of living."

diethylstilbestrol (DES). A type of synthetic estrogen used in the 1940s through to the 1960s as a growth hormone to fatten meat-producing animals. It was also given to pregnant women to prevent miscarriages but is now banned because it was found to cause both cancer and birth abnormalities.

diuretic. A substance (medication or food) that rids the body of excess fluid by increasing the flow of urine.

edema. Swelling of tissues in the body caused by an abnormal accumulation of fluid.

electrolyte(s). A large category of substances—which include sodium, potassium, calcium, magnesium, chloride and bicarbonate—whose water solution will carry an electric current. Cells use electrolytes to transmit electrical impulses (nerve impulses, muscle contractions) across themselves and to other cells. These chemicals are essential in many bodily processes, such as fluid balance, nerve conduction, muscle function (including heartbeat), blood clotting and pH balance.

endocrine disruptor. An environmental poison that mimics, blocks or otherwise disrupts the normal function of hormones. It is an exogenous (coming from outside the body) substance that changes endocrine function and can cause adverse developmental and reproductive effects in living organisms and their offspring, as well as being a potential carcinogen in the environment. Examples include pesticides, insecticides, herbicides, fungicides, plastics, solvents and heavy metals.

endocrine system. The entire collection of glands that produce and release hormones; together these glands and hormones influence almost every cell, organ and function of the body. The system as a whole communicates through the blood vessels and lymphatic system. Hormones are sent from one gland to another, or to a remote tissue, creating some effect. The characteristic feature of the endocrine glands is that they are ductless (without ducts). Because the liver does have a duct (bile duct connection to the small intestine), it is not considered a true endocrine gland even though it produces a hormone. This system is the body's main communication system. The term *endocrine* is derived from the Greek words *endon*, "within," and *krinein*, "to separate."

enzyme. A protein substance produced by all living plants and animals that both causes and greatly increases the speed of chemical reactions. Found in every organ of the body, enzymes cause specific chemical changes without being used up or chemically altered themselves. Enzymes are known to catalyze about 4,000 biochemical reactions. For instance, the liver produces enzymes to break down toxic chemicals into harmless substances; other enzymes change starches, proteins and sugars into material the body can digest; blood clotting is another example. Without enzymes, chemical reactions would be very slow.

epinephrine. See **adrenaline**.

estrogen. A general name for the female sex hormone produced by the ovaries. There are three main naturally occurring estrogens in women: estradiol, estriol and estrone. These are responsible for the female characteristics, menstrual cycle, and changes of the uterus and breasts; they also provide the fat layer around the female body. Derived from the Greek *oistros*, "mad desire," and *genēs*, "born."

fat (dietary). Provides essential fatty acids for growth and development of body tissue, as well as fat-soluble vitamins. Essential fatty acids are fats that must come from the diet—flax or fish oil, nuts, olives, avocados, vegetables (or their oils) and seeds. The body can also make some of the fats it needs from carbohydrates.

fibromyalgia. An inflammatory condition that affects many muscles, joints and connective tissues in the body.

genetically modified organisms (GMOs). Organisms that have had their genes manipulated (1) to introduce new, or alter existing, characteristics, or (2) to produce a new protein or enzyme. Genetic modification produces crops that carry certain traits such as resistance to insect damage and herbicides (chemical weed killers).

gland. An organ or structure whose secretions include hormones, mucus and sweat. Derived from the Latin *glans*, meaning "acorn."

glucagon. The opposing hormone to insulin, glucagon raises blood sugar and is a fat-burning hormone. It helps regulate blood sugar between meals and is stimulated by proteins and intense exercise.

glucose. The simplest form of sugar and carbohydrate. The body uses hormones to change body proteins into sugar and stores glucose in the liver and muscles as glycogen.

glutamic acid. A non-essential amino acid that occurs widely in plant and animal tissue and is used by the body to build proteins. It is supplied by most food sources of protein. Glutamate, a salt of glutamic acid, has a stimulating effect on the central nervous system. Monosodium glutamate (MSG) is a form of glutamic acid used as a flavor enhancer.

gluten. The protein part of wheat.

GMO. See **genetically modified organisms**.

growth hormone (GH). A fat-burning, lean-muscle-building hormone that contributes to growth. GH rebuilds body tissue, including joints, bones and muscles; it also builds up cartilage and collagen. It is an anti-aging hormone. Growth hormone works through the liver; it regulates fuel between meals and is active during the sleep cycle.

hormone. A chemical message that originates in an organ or gland and is sent through the blood or lymph to another part of the body, triggering an increase or decrease in function. Hormones are made from cholesterol, amino acids, fatty acids and protein. Functions include burning fat, storing fat, the regulation of sleep cycles, blood pressure, cholesterol levels and hair growth, and changes in the menstrual cycle. Hormones also control the reproductive cycle of virtually all multicellular organisms. There are several hundred hormones and each one has a different action and effect. Environmental chemicals and toxins can also mimic, block, alter and confuse hormones. Derived from the Greek *hormon*, from *horman*, "to set in motion."

hormone-free animal products. Products from animals raised without added hormones.

hormone receptor. A sensor tissue in the body that receives hormonal messages. Receptors can be on the cells' surface or within the cells.

hormone replacement therapy (HRT). A synthetic blend of the hormone estrogen and progestin (a synthetic form of progesterone), used to replace hormones the female body no longer produces after menopause. Studies show that side effects include stroke, cancer, and possibly heart disease. There are conflicting data on whether HRT is beneficial or harmful to the heart.

hydrogenate. To combine a fluid oil with hydrogen in order to produce a solid fat.

hydrolyze. To subject to hydrolysis—a chemical process in which a substance reacts to water so as to be changed from one thing into another, such as a starch to glucose or a fat into fatty acids or a protein into its component amino acids. In protein powders, hydrolyzing is a form of predigesting the protein to make it absorb more easily when eaten. Hydrolyzed proteins are also proteins from certain foods that have been treated with an acid or enzyme and are then used in the same manner as MSG in products such as canned vegetables, soups and processed meats.

hypothalamus. A master gland in the brain that controls homeostasis (the body's ability to adapt to environmental changes and maintain normal stability of its internal functions—temperature, blood sugar, blood pressure, etc.).

hypothesis. A tentative explanation for an observation, phenomenon or scientific problem that needs to be tested by further investigation.

immune system. The body's defense mechanism against disease, infection and foreign substances. It is made up of highly specialized cells, tissues and organs, with a circulatory system separate from blood vessels, all of which work together to protect the body. The special circulatory system carries lymph, a transparent fluid containing white blood cells whose function is to seek out and destroy the organisms or substances that cause disease. See also **lymphatic system**.

insulin. Hormone produced by the pancreas that lowers blood sugar after meals to maintain normal blood sugars and prevent high blood sugar levels. Insulin will cause the cells to absorb sugar as fuel and will convert the rest to fat and cholesterol.

insulin-like growth factor (IGF). Hormone made by the liver that regulates blood sugars between meals. It releases stored sugar and fat, maintaining blood glucose at a normal level. Insulin and IGF work in tandem to keep blood sugars in balance.

insulin resistance. A condition where the insulin receptors on the surface of the cells won't let insulin be accepted, causing the pancreas to secrete higher amounts of insulin. When the body cells resist or do not respond even to high levels of insulin, glucose builds up in the blood creating a type 2 diabetes situation.

iodized salt. Salt that has iodine added to it. Used primarily to prevent thyroid problems.

ion. An atom or group of atoms that are normally electrically neutral and become electrically charged during a chemical reaction.

isolate. A dry powder food ingredient—such as soy protein isolate or whey protein isolate—that has been separated, or isolated, from the other components of the soybean, whey, etc., making it 90 to 95 percent protein and nearly carbohydrate- and fat-free.

ketosis. Ketones are a normal byproduct of fat metabolism (the breaking down of fat into energy). When ketones are in the urine, it means the body is breaking down fat. There are two types of ketosis: (1) *dietary ketosis*, which is the body's normal reaction when a person consumes primarily or only fat and protein, thus forcing the body to burn fat; (2) *ketoacidosis*, which is a dangerous condition for diabetics and is considered a disease, where the blood pH becomes overly acidic due to extremely high blood glucose, and ketones are produced by the body to provide the fuel necessary for life, since the sugar cannot be utilized because of the diabetes.

lactic acid. A waste product of sugar metabolism. The body generates lactic acid when stored sugar is burned from the muscles and liver. The body can also use lactic acid as a fuel source, burning it in a way similar to the way it burns a sugar fuel. The body will utilize sugar and lactic acid as fuel before it uses fat as fuel.

lecithin. A substance that helps break down fats and cholesterol. Lecithin is present in eggs and other foods that contain fat. It is considered anti-cholesterol.

lymphatic system. A major part of the immune system, it helps defend the body against viruses, bacteria and fungi that can cause illnesses. Its three main functions are maintaining fluid balance in the body, immunity, and the absorption and transport of fatty acids from the small intestine to the blood. The system is made up of a network of lymphatic vessels, which carry lymph (a clear, watery fluid containing the disease-fighting white blood cells as well as salts, glucose and other substances) throughout the body; lymph nodes—small masses of tissue located along the lymph vessels, which house a type of white blood cell and filter out destroyed microorganisms; and lymph organs, including the bone marrow, spleen, thymus gland and tonsils. The word *lymph* comes from the French *lymphe*, from Latin *lympha*, meaning "clear water." See also **immune system**.

metabolic rate. The rate at which the body utilizes energy. This rate is controlled by hormones. The thyroid gland is a very important factor in metabolic rate.

metabolism. The sum of the physical and chemical changes that occur in the body, necessary for the maintenance of life. Examples are the breaking down of food to produce energy and the utilization of that energy to perform vital life functions; and the breakdown of fat and stored sugar, yielding fuel to power other bodily activities. Metabolism involves two processes: (1) the building up of tissue (anabolism), as occurs in bone or muscle growth; and (2) the breaking down of tissue (catabolism), as in the release of fat from the reserves or the breakdown of muscle tissue after exercise. Metabolism is influenced by hormones. The term derives from the Greek word *metabolē*, "change," + *-ism*, meaning "the condition of."

mitochondria. Very small, usually rod-like structures found in the cells, which act as energy factories to regulate metabolism. Fat and sugar are turned into energy by the mitochondria, and the thyroid gland controls their number and size.

myxedema. A skin and tissue disorder caused by an extreme deficiency of thyroid hormone. It is characterized by dry, thickening skin and a swelling of the skin and other tissues, particularly around the eyes, lips and nose. The swelling is not a true form of fat, but rather a waste-like substance that accumulates between the cells. Fluid is trapped as well. Because of its sponge-like nature, the excess fluid remains immobile, and the edema is non-pitting—that is, if pressure is applied to the skin, it does not result in a persistent indentation. Derived from the Greek *myxa*, "mucus" or "slime," and *oidēma*, "swelling."

nitrates. Refers to sodium nitrate—a chemical used to preserve and color food, especially meat and fish products; implicated in the formation of suspected carcinogens.

organic. 1. Grown with only animal or vegetable fertilizers, such as manure, bone meal or compost, and without the use of chemical fertilizers, pesticides, fungicides, herbicides or insecticides, or genetically modified organisms or products produced by or from GMOs. Organic meat, poultry, eggs and dairy products come from animals that are given no antibiotics or growth hormones. **2.** Plant-based; derived from living organisms. Plants take rocks from the soil—calcium carbonate, iron ore, copper—and change these inorganic minerals to plant-based (organic) minerals, making the bonds between the molecules weaker and thus easier for the body to break down. [Note: These definitions apply to the use of *organic* within this book. Further definitions can be found in a dictionary.]

parasympathetic nervous system. Part of the nervous system that controls largely automatic processes such as digestion, breathing and heart rate. Sometimes called the "rest and digest" system, it acts together with the sympathetic nervous system to conserve the body's energy by slowing the heart rate, increasing intestinal and gland activity, and relaxing muscles in the stomach and intestinal tract, particularly after the fight-or-flight response is activated by the sympathetic nervous system. See also **sympathetic nervous system**.

pH. A symbol used (with a number) to indicate acidity or alkalinity. It represents the concentration of hydrogen ions in a given solution. On the pH scale, values range from 0 to 14. A pH of 7 is considered neutral. Pure water has a pH of 7. Substances with a pH value above 7 are alkaline; those with a pH below 7 are acidic. The term derives from German: *p* stands for *Potenz*, meaning "potency" or "power," and *H* is the symbol for hydrogen, the ion that determines acidity or alkalinity.

pituitary. A gland in the brain that acts as a relay between the hypothalamus and other glands (ovaries, adrenals, liver, thyroid and testes).

polycystic ovarian syndrome (PCOS). A condition where multiple small cysts form in the ovaries (*poly* means "many"), related to the ovary's failure to release an egg. PCOS can create facial hair, weight gain, insulin resistance and a disruption in the menstrual cycle.

protein. One of the three types of nutrients used by the body as energy sources, the other two being carbohydrate and fat. Its building blocks are amino acids. The body's cells are composed of 50 percent protein. Protein is needed for growth and development and is used by the body to make muscles, organs, glands, skin, bone, hair, nails, blood and the immune system; even body fluids (except bile and urine) contain protein. See also **amino acids**.

Ragland's test. A blood pressure test used to indicate the general health of the adrenal glands, which provides information on how the adrenals respond to stress. The blood pressure is first taken when a person has been lying down for a few minutes. It is then taken a second time, immediately after the person stands up. In a normal reading, the top number (systolic) is from 6 to 10 points higher when the person is standing than when he or she is lying down. A rise of 0 to 5 points indicates a borderline adrenal problem, while a drop gives a relative indication of diminished adrenal function.

saccharin. The oldest-known artificial sweetener, it is a white crystalline powder produced from coal tar, having a taste about 500 times sweeter than cane sugar but with a slightly bitter metallic aftertaste. The sodium or calcium salt of saccharin is widely used as a calorie-free sweetener in special dietary foods and beverages and to improve the taste of pharmaceuticals, toothpaste and other toiletries; it is also used as a sugar substitute in diabetic diets.

serotonin. A hormone found in the brain, blood and digestive tract, which allows nerve cells throughout the body to communicate and interact with each other. It helps smooth muscles to contract, such as the abdominal muscles that aid digestion, and also plays a part in regulating the expansion and contraction of blood vessels, assisting in the clotting of blood to close a wound. Some of the body's serotonin is produced by the adrenal glands, and its presence in the body creates a sense of well-being or comfort.

Splenda. Also known as sucralose, it is an artificial sweetener derived from chlorinated sucrose (table sugar). It is 320 to 1,000 times sweeter than sucrose. While there are no long-term human studies for sucralose, animal studies have shown shrunken thymus glands (up to 40 percent shrinkage), enlarged liver and kidneys, atrophy of lymph follicles in the spleen and thymus, reduced growth rate, decreased red blood cell count, aborted pregnancy, decreased placental and fetal body weights, and diarrhea.

steroids. Any of numerous natural or synthetic fat-soluble compounds, including many hormones, body components (e.g., cholesterol, bile acids, and the adrenal and sex hormones) and drugs. Steroid hormones such as cortisol or cortisone are anti-inflammatory hormones produced by the adrenal glands.

stevia. A herb or shrub of the same family as sunflowers, its extracts have up to 300 times the sweetness of sugar.

sulfite. A type of food preservative, often found in wines, dried fruits and dried potato products, and sometimes added to bottled juices, pickles and other food items.

sympathetic nervous system. Part of the nervous system that prepares the body for physical action, emergency or sudden stress. The heartbeat accelerates, blood sugar rises, perspiration occurs, digestion is slowed, blood flow to the skin is decreased, and arteries are dilated, increasing blood flow to the muscles. This process is known as the body's fight-or-flight response. See also **parasympathetic nervous system**.

synthetic vitamins. Vitamins manufactured from chemicals (mostly coal-tar products) as compared with whole vitamin complexes found in nature that come from plant and animal sources. They are isolated parts of the vitamins that occur naturally in food, and they not only cannot perform the same functions in the body as natural whole vitamin complexes but in many cases can be harmful to the system.

systolic. The blood pressure when the heart is contracting. In a blood pressure reading, the systolic pressure is the first number recorded. For example, if the reading is 120/80, the top number of 120 is the systolic measurement. By "120" is meant 120 millimeters of mercury. This number measures the pressure against the blood vessel walls when the heart is pumping blood to the organs. Derived from the Greek *systolē*, from *systellein*, "to draw together." See also **diastolic**.

testosterone. A steroid hormone from the androgen group. Testosterone is secreted primarily in the testicles of males and the ovaries of females, although small amounts are secreted by the adrenal glands. It is the principal male sex hormone. In both males and females, it plays key roles in health and well-being. Examples include enhanced libido, energy, immune function, and protection against osteoporosis.

trans fats. Also known as trans fatty acids and hydrogenated or partially hydrogenated fats, these are man-made or processed fats, produced by adding hydrogen gas to a liquid fat or oil to make it thicker or more solid. This increases its shelf life, as it is less likely to spoil. Hydrogenating the oil in peanut butter, for instance, gives the product a creamy consistency and prevents the oil from rising to the top. However, trans fats are very hard on the liver, and consuming them can contribute to an increase in total cholesterol as well as a drop in the good cholesterol. They also increase the risk of heart disease. Trans fats can be found in numerous foods, including commercially prepared baked goods, some commercially fried foods, packaged snacks, cakes, cookies, crackers, peanut butter, stick margarine and vegetable shortening. Harvard School of Public Health estimates there are 30,000 American deaths each year from eating trans fats, making these fats silent killers.*

triglycerides. Blood fats.

virus. A portion of genetic material wrapped in protein. Viruses can reproduce only by invading and taking over other cells because they lack the cellular machinery for self-reproduction. They are parasitic, which means they live off the energy from other cells. People become susceptible to viruses when their resistance is lowered. Viruses can be sent into remission (inactivation).

vitamins. A group of compounds needed in small amounts by the body to maintain health and normal functioning. Vitamins are obtained from food, and some are made by the body. They are not used by the body as fuel but rather as cofactors and regulators of cell function. (A *cofactor* is an accessory substance that must be present for a particular biological reaction to occur.) Derived from the Latin *vita*, which means "life," + *amine*, because vitamins were originally thought to contain amino acids.

vitamins K and J. Vitamin K is a fat-soluble vitamin that promotes blood clotting; vitamin J is the anti-pneumonia factor. Normally these two vitamins work synergistically with vitamin C.

---

* *Source:* Harvard Medical School (2004).

References

For complete documentation on the authors and publications cited below, refer to the bibliography on pages 347–49.

CHAPTER 2: *The 7 Principles of Fat Burning*

1. Netter, *CIBA Collection of Medical Illustrations*, Vol. 4, 101.
   Bacon and Di Bisceglie, *Liver Disease*, 24.
2. Gillette, Bullough, and Melby, "Postexercise Energy Expenditure," 347–60.
   Schuenke, Mikat, and McBride, "Post-Exercise Oxygen Consumption," 411–17.

CHAPTER 3: *Hormones and Your Body Shape*

1. Netter, *CIBA Collection of Medical Illustrations*, Vol. 4, 121.
2. U.S. EPA, "What Is Endocrine Disruption?"
   https://www.epa.gov/endocrine-disruption/what-endocrine-disruption.
3. Berkson, *Hormone Deception*, 218.
4. Klaassen, *Casarett & Doull's Toxicology*, 16.

CHAPTER 5: *The Adrenal Type*

1. Guyton, *Textbook of Medical Physiology*, 916.
2. Netter, *CIBA Collection of Medical Illustrations*, Vol. 4, 85.
3. Guyton, *Textbook of Medical Physiology*, 916.
4. Guyton, *Textbook of Medical Physiology*, 822.
   Guyton, *Textbook of Medical Physiology*, 823.

5. Guyton, *Textbook of Medical Physiology*, 817.
   Guyton, *Textbook of Medical Physiology*, 914.
6. Netter, *CIBA Collection of Medical Illustrations*, Vol. 4, 86.
7. Netter, *CIBA Collection of Medical Illustrations*, Vol. 4, 87.
8. Netter, *CIBA Collection of Medical Illustrations*, Vol. 4, 87.
9. Netter, *CIBA Collection of Medical Illustrations*, Vol. 4, 85.
10. Netter, *CIBA Collection of Medical Illustrations*, Vol. 4, 86.
11. Netter, *CIBA Collection of Medical Illustrations*, Vol. 4, 87.
12. Guyton, *Textbook of Medical Physiology*, 917.

CHAPTER 7: *The Thyroid Type*

1. Guyton, *Textbook of Medical Physiology*, 816.
2. Lee, *About Menopause*, 147.
3. Shomon, *Living Well with Hypothyroidism*, 268.
4. Colborn, Dumanoski, and Myers, *Our Stolen Future*, 40.
5. Guyton, *Textbook of Medical Physiology*, 907.

CHAPTER 8: *The Liver Type*

1. Bacon and Di Bisceglie, *Liver Disease*, 21.
2. Netter, *CIBA Collection of Medical Illustrations*, Vol. 3, 84.
   Netter, *CIBA Collection of Medical Illustrations*, Vol. 3, 97.
3. Netter, *CIBA Collection of Medical Illustrations*, Vol. 4, 71.
4. Netter, *CIBA Collection of Medical Illustrations*, Vol. 3, 70.
5. Netter, *CIBA Collection of Medical Illustrations*, Vol. 3, 71.
6. Netter, *CIBA Collection of Medical Illustrations*, Vol. 4, 156.
7. Bacon and Di Bisceglie, *Liver Disease*, 24–28.
8. Netter, *CIBA Collection of Medical Illustrations*, Vol. 3, 42.
9. Netter, *CIBA Collection of Medical Illustrations*, Vol. 4, 212.
10. Faigin, *Natural Hormonal Enhancement*, 201.
11. Faigin, *Natural Hormonal Enhancement*, 6.
12. Faigin, *Natural Hormonal Enhancement*, 8.

CHAPTER 9: *The 10 Fat-Burning Triggers and Blockers*

Trigger #1—The Absence of Sugar

1. Guyton, *Textbook of Medical Physiology*, 823.
2. Guyton, *Textbook of Medical Physiology*, 819.
   Guyton, *Textbook of Medical Physiology*, 820.
   Guyton, *Textbook of Medical Physiology*, 822.
   Guyton, *Textbook of Medical Physiology*, 926.
   Guyton, *Textbook of Medical Physiology*, 930.
3. Guyton, *Textbook of Medical Physiology*, 822.
   Guyton, *Textbook of Medical Physiology*, 824.
   Guyton, *Textbook of Medical Physiology*, 927.
   Guyton, *Textbook of Medical Physiology*, 930.
4. Guyton, *Textbook of Medical Physiology*, 823.
   Guyton, *Textbook of Medical Physiology*, 931.
   Griffin and Ojeda, *Endocrine Physiology*, 396.
5. Faigin, *Natural Hormonal Enhancement*, 239.
6. Guyton, *Textbook of Medical Physiology*, 930.
   Guyton, *Textbook of Medical Physiology*, 932.
7. Guyton, *Textbook of Medical Physiology*, 930.
   Guyton, *Textbook of Medical Physiology*, 931.

Trigger #3—Protein

8. Guyton, *Textbook of Medical Physiology*, 889.
   Guyton, *Textbook of Medical Physiology*, 932.
9. Guyton, *Textbook of Medical Physiology*, 862.

Trigger #4—Fats

10. Guyton, *Textbook of Medical Physiology*, 825.
    Griffin and Ojeda, *Endocrine Physiology*, 404.
11. Lewis et al., "Effect of Diet Composition," 160–70.
12. Netter, *CIBA Collection of Medical Illustrations*, Vol. 3, 52.
    Colorado State University, "Cholecystokinin,"
    http://www.vivo.colostate.edu./hbooks/pathphys/endocrine/gi/cck.html.
13. Guyton, *Textbook of Medical Physiology*, 822.
    Netter, *CIBA Collection of Medical Illustrations*, Vol. 3, 37.
    Yancy et al., "Low-Carbohydrate, Ketogenic Diet," 769–77.
    Achten and Jeukendrup, "Optimizing Fat Oxidation," 723.

Trigger #6—Gland Destroyers

14. Bacon and Di Bisceglie, *Liver Disease*, 24.
    Bacon and Di Bisceglie, *Liver Disease*, 25.
15. Lane et al., "Caffeine Effects," 320–36.

Trigger #8—Exercise

16. Faigin, *Natural Hormonal Enhancement*, 238–40.
17. Faigin, *Natural Hormonal Enhancement*, 242.
18. Nicklas, *Endurance Exercise and Adipose Tissue*, 5.
19. Guyton, *Textbook of Medical Physiology*, 824.
    Guyton, *Textbook of Medical Physiology*, 889, fig. 75-5.
    Guyton, *Textbook of Medical Physiology*, 930.
    Guyton, *Textbook of Medical Physiology*, 932.

Trigger #9—Stress

20. Guyton, *Textbook of Medical Physiology*, 918.
    Netter, *CIBA Collection of Medical Illustrations*, Vol. 4, 85.

Trigger #10—Sleep

21. Guyton, *Textbook of Medical Physiology*, 889.
22. Netter, *CIBA Collection of Medical Illustrations*, Vol. 4, 87.
23. Faigin, *Natural Hormonal Enhancement*, 201.

CHAPTER 17: *Exercising for Your Body Type*

1. Guyton, *Textbook of Medical Physiology*, 932.
2. Schuenke, Mikat, and McBride,
   "Post-Exercise Oxygen Consumption," 411–17.

Bibliography

Achten, Juul, and Asker E. Jeukendrup. "Optimizing Fat Oxidation through Exercise and Diet." *Nutrition* 20, nos. 7/8 (2004): 716–27.

Bacon, Bruce R., and Adrian M. Di Bisceglie, eds. *Liver Disease: Diagnosis and Management.* Philadelphia: Churchill Livingstone, 2000.

Berkson, D. Lindsey. *Hormone Deception.* Chicago: Contemporary Books, 2000.

Colborn, Theo, Dianne Dumanoski, and John Peterson Myers. *Our Stolen Future.* New York: Plume, 1997.

Colorado State University. "Pathophysiology of the Endocrine System: Gastrointestinal Hormones: Cholecystokinin." *Hypertexts for Biomedical Sciences.* http://www.vivo.colostate.edu./hbooks/pathphys/endocrine/gi/cck.html.

Crickenberger, Roger G., and Roy E. Carawan. "Using Food Processing By-Products for Animal Feed." *Water Quality and Waste Management*, North Carolina Cooperative Extension Service, 1996.

Diabetes in Control. "390 Drugs That Can Affect Blood Glucose Levels." March 4, 2016. http://www.diabetesincontrol.com/drugs-that-can-affect-blood-glucose-levels/.

Faigin, Rob. *Natural Hormonal Enhancement.* Cedar Mountain, NC: Extique, 2000.

George Mateljan Foundation. *The World's Healthiest Foods.* http://www.whfoods.org/foodstoc.php.

Gillette, C. A., R. C. Bullough, and C. L. Melby. "Postexercise Energy Expenditure in Response to Acute Aerobic or Resistive Exercise." *Int J Sport Nutr 4*, no. 4 (1994): 347–60.

Griffin, James E., and Sergio R. Ojeda, eds. *Textbook of Endocrine Physiology.* 4th ed. New York: Oxford University Press, 2000.

Guyton, Arthur C. *Textbook of Medical Physiology.* 7th ed. Philadelphia: W. B. Saunders, 1986.

Harvard Medical School. "Trans Fat: Watch Out, It Isn't So Transparent!" Harvard Health Publications, March 2004. http://www.health.harvard.edu/press_releases/trans_fat.

Kirby, Alex. "Waste 'Was Fed to UK Cattle.'" *BBC News,* October 27, 1999. http://news.bbc.co.uk/1/hi/sci/tech/486421.stm.

Klaassen, Curtis D., ed. *Casarett & Doull's Toxicology: The Basic Science of Poisons.* 6th ed. New York: McGraw-Hill, 2001.

Lane, J. D., R. A. Adcock, R. B. Williams, and C. M. Kuhn. "Caffeine Effects on Cardiovascular and Neuroendocrine Responses to Acute Psychosocial Stress and Their Relationship to Level of Habitual Caffeine Consumption." *Psychosom Med* 52, no. 3 (1990): 320–36.

Lee, John R. *What Your Doctor May Not Tell You about Menopause.* With Virginia Hopkins. New York: Warner Books, 1996.

Lewis, S. B., J. D. Wallin, J. P. Kane, and J. E. Gerich. "Effect of Diet Composition on Metabolic Adaptations to Hypocaloric Nutrition: Comparison of High Carbohydrate and High Fat Isocaloric Diets." *Am J Clin Nutr* 30, no. 2 (1977): 160–70.

Netter, Frank H. *The CIBA Collection of Medical Illustrations.* Vol. 3, *Digestive System,* Part III: *Liver, Biliary Tract and Pancreas.* 2nd ed. New York: CIBA Pharmaceutical, 1972.

———. *The CIBA Collection of Medical Illustrations.* Vol. 4, *Endocrine System and Selected Metabolic Diseases.* New York: CIBA Pharmaceutical, 1970.

Nicklas, Barbara, ed. *Endurance Exercise and Adipose Tissue.* Boca Raton, FL: CRC Press, 2002.

Research Consortium Sustainable Animal Production. "Animal Nutrition: Resources and New Challenges: Summary." http://agriculture.de/acms1/conf6/ws8sum.htm.

Schuenke, Mark D., Richard P. Mikat, and Jeffrey M. McBride. "Effect of an Acute Period of Resistance Exercise on Excess Post-Exercise Oxygen Consumption: Implications for Body Mass Management." *Eur J Appl Physiol* 86, no. 5 (2002): 411–17.

Shomon, Mary J. *Living Well with Hypothyroidism: What Your Doctor Doesn't Tell You . . . That You Need to Know.* New York: Avon Books, 2000.

Stitt, Paul A. *Beating the Food Giants.* Manitowoc, WI: Natural Press, 1993.

U.S. Department of Health & Human Services. "Adverse Reactions Associated with Aspartame Consumption." HFS-728. Chief, Epidemiology Branch, April 1, 1993.

U.S. Department of Health & Human Services and U.S. Environmental Protection Agency. "What You Need to Know about Mercury in Fish and Shellfish: 2004 EPA and FDA Advice for Women Who Might Become Pregnant, Women Who Are Pregnant, Nursing Mothers, Young Children." EPA-823-R-04-005, March 2004.

U.S. EPA (U.S. Environmental Protection Agency). "What Is Endocrine Disruption?" https://www.epa.gov/endocrine-disruption/what-endocrine-disruption.

Yancy, William S., Jr., Maren K. Olsen, John R. Guyton, Ronna P. Bakst, and Eric C. Westman. "A Low-Carbohydrate, Ketogenic Diet versus a Low-Fat Diet to Treat Obesity and Hyperlipidemia." *Ann Intern Med* 140, no. 10 (2004): 769–77.

Resources

Dr. Berg's Products

You can order these products from the Health & Wellness Center by going online to www.DrBerg.com or by calling 1-800-816-8184 during normal business hours. For support, email DrBerg@drberg.com.

Product List

Adrenal Night Formula / Dr. Berg's Sleep Aid

This nutritional support addresses the quality of your sleep by reducing adrenal stress. With a combination of adrenal-relaxing nutrients and the addition of adrenal-supporting vitamins, it can help you get to sleep quickly for seven to eight hours of uninterrupted quality sleep.

Adrenal Day Formula / Dr. Berg's Adrenal & Cortisol Relief

This product is designed to reduce stress and keep your body in a relaxed state. If you have a low tolerance for stress, excessive brain chatter or an inability to relax, you will benefit from this remedy.

Gallbladder Formula

This formula is a combination of digestive nutrients to support the gallbladder, stomach and pancreas. It includes purified bile salts, digestive enzymes, Digest Formula and herbs to help optimize your digestion.

Apple Cider Vinegar Plus / Digest Formula

This will assist in supporting your stomach by enhancing your acids. Use it to counteract indigestion, acid reflux or GERD.

Estrogen Balance with DIM

This product targets premenopause and menopause symptoms. It contains key nutrients to support estrogen dominance, using a highly concentrated cruciferous extract (called DIM) and other hormone-supportive ingredients.

Dr. Berg's Instant Kale Shake

This shake is an excellent meal replacement, containing pea protein and kale with no added sugar.

Dr. Berg's Meal Replacement Shake with MCTs*

This new meal-replacement formula contains pea protein and MCTs from coconut oil. It has a chocolate-brownie flavor with an amazing texture similar to a chocolate milkshake. MCTs can help support fat burning.

Dr. Berg's Organic Cruciferous Superfood

This product contains both organic cruciferous vegetables and additional superfoods to help support a healthy liver and estrogen balance.

---

* MCTs are medium-chain triglycerides. These special types of fats assist in fat burning and are less stressful on the gallbladder.

Dr. Berg's Adrenal Body Type Kit

This kit contains four products—Dr. Berg's targeted nutrient blends designed to help support the Adrenal body type. Together these provide the most complete overall solution for the Adrenal body type.

Dr. Berg's Self-Massage Tool

This device is used to reduce stress and enhance your sleep. It comes with an instruction manual for easy use.

Dr. Berg's Raw Wheat Grass Juice Powder with Kamut (Lemon)

This new product is Dr. Berg's ultimate in concentrated greens, containing both raw organic wheat-grass juice powder and organic Kamut wheat-grass juice powder. Kamut is an ancient wheat grain that contains higher levels of protein and nutrients than most wheat. We added natural lemon flavor with a touch of stevia. Our regular Raw Wheat Grass Juice Powder is also available.

Dr. Berg's Trace Minerals

This product contains plant-based trace minerals in a liquid. Trace minerals are usually missing in our soils and our foods. These micronutrients assist protein formation in the body at the DNA level as well as the muscle, bone and organ levels.

Dr. Berg's Sea Kelp (from Iceland)

This high-quality sea kelp from Iceland is 100 percent organic. It can help support a healthy thyroid as well as nourishing both female organs and the male prostate gland.

Other Resources

Dr. Berg's Video Tip of the Week

If you would like to receive Dr. Berg's email video tips of the week, go to www.DrBerg.com and sign up.

Dr. Berg's Body Type Quiz

Go to www.DrBerg.com to take Dr. Berg's Body Type Quiz.

Advanced Evaluation Questionnaire

Take the quiz by going to www.DrBerg.com/evaluation.

Dr. Berg's Acupressure Techniques

For more information on Dr. Berg's acupressure techniques, go to www.DrBerg.com. The do-it-yourself version is in chapter 16.

Dr. Berg's Exclusive Membership Site

This is Dr. Berg's online do-it-yourself get-healthy program. It targets the Adrenal body type, yet it is helpful for all body types. Loaded with over 200 videos, this site offers a complete education in getting your body super healthy.

Dr. Berg's Health Coaching Training

This online digital training is for those who want to be certified in Dr. Berg's health coaching.

Dr. Berg's YouTube Channel

Watch Dr. Berg's daily videos at https://www.youtube.com/user/drericberg123. You can also subscribe to receive Dr. Berg's daily videos. Currently Dr. Berg has over 78 million views, with more than 600,000 subscribers.

Enzymes to Help with Digestion

If you have a sensitivity to certain vegetables or beans that results in uncomfortable bloating, you can order the specific enzymes you need from this website: http://www.bean-zyme.com/.

The Future of Food Video

http://www.thefutureoffood.com/

Dr. Berg's New Frozen Dessert

Finally, there's a delicious treat that is both pleasurable and healthy. With less than 1 gram of sugar per serving, Dr. Berg's *Kebby's Frozen Dessert* will satisfy that hunger for ice cream. This product is keto-friendly, lactose-free and made with creamy coconut oil. Go to www.DrBerg.com for more information.

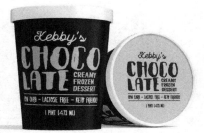
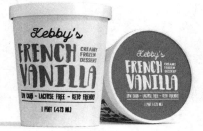

Index

Page numbers in italics refer to charts or illustrations.

A

Acid reflux, 129, 167, 168, 169, 352

Acne, 49, 157

Acupressure, 146, 162, 231–244
  Injury Technique, 226, *226*
  Liver Technique, 199–200, *200*, 229
  for stress, 197–198, 228, 231
  Thyroid Technique, 204
  See also Massage tool

Adrenal body type, *8*, *9*, 10, 43–52, *45*
  acupressure for, 197, 228, 229
  bladder issues, 52
  blood alkalinity, 188
  causes of, 65–66
  cortisol and, 47
  exercise effects, 21, 53, 55, 159, 245,
      247, 254
  exercise for, 20, 53, 159, 198, 245,
      247, 257
  exercise plan, 263–267
  facial characteristics, 47, *48*
  fats, 196
  food cravings, 60
  nutrients for, 196–197

pH, 197
proteins and, 127, 196
salt needed for, 319
stages, 47, *47*
stimulants, 59, 66
stress-reducing techniques for, 197–198
sugar and, 48
symptoms (list), 66–67

Adrenal glands, 10, 25, 43–44, *43*, 64–65
  autoimmune conditions and, 202
  blockers, 207
  blood pressure and, 56–57
  blood sugar levels and, 62, *63*
  caffeine and, 207
  functional deficiency problems, 59–63
  immune system and, 63–64
  ovaries and, 74
  oxygen levels and, 55
  stress and, 58–59, 228
  thyroid autoimmunity and, 87

Adrenal hormones, 13, 65
  beets and, 141
  blood pressure and, 56–57
  calcium and, 49–50
  celery effects on, 148, 316
  circadian rhythms and, 50–51, *51*

deficiency, 52–57
ear ringing and, 57
functions, 44
immune system and, 44
potassium loss and, 49–50
pthalides and, 148, 316
stress and, 50, 58, 202, 247

Adrenaline, 34, 139, 247

Aerobic exercise, 145–146, 245, 250
anaerobic vs., 247
benefits, 263
duration and rest periods, *265*, 266
examples of, *265*
mixing with anaerobic, 266
routine, 264–266
sugar-burning to fat-burning ratios, *264*
weight training, 264
See also Exercise

Agave nectar, 118, 171, 205

Alcohol. *See* Beverages

Alkalinity, bodily. *See* pH

Allergies, 64, 170, 177, 312–313
symptom of pH imbalance, 188
See also Food sensitivities

Almond butter, 128, 158, 173

Almond flour, *211*, 306

Amino acids, 6, 128, 151, 314
essential, 6, 153
food sources, 128, 216, 217

Anaerobic exercise, 145, 245, 254, 256, 258
aerobic vs., 247
drawbacks, 263
durations, 261, *261*
factors in, *260*, 261
hormones and, 258–259, *259*
mixing with aerobic, 266
optimum, *262*
rest periods, *261*
routine, 259
variables, *262*
weight training, 264

workout examples, 259–260, *260*
See also Exercise

Animal feeds, 90, 209–210

Ankles, swollen, 61, *61*, 102, 105, 144, 322

Antibiotics, 104, 140, 169
animal use, 209
in foods, 32, 107, 210, *212*

Antioxidants, 116, 323
ascorbic acid, 65, 197

Appetite suppressants, 13, 19, 139

Apple cider vinegar, 159, 187, 322
to balance pH, 197
for bloating, 167
candida and, 104
drink, 171, 187–188, *189–190, 213*
insulin function and, 187, 204
kidney stones and, 322
as salad dressing, 177
stomach acidity and, 204
vegetable wash, 32

Apples, 117, 177–178, 205

Apricots, 178, 313

Arginine, 128

Arteries, clogged. *See* Atherosclerosis

Arteriosclerosis, 50, 57

Arthritis, 12, 50, 100, 101

Artificial sweeteners. *See* Sugar substitutes

Ascites, 94–96, *96*

Asthma, 56, 64

Atherosclerosis, 108

Attention deficit disorder (ADD), 83

Autoimmune conditions, 202
adrenals and, 64, 87

Avocados, 160, 174
amino acids in, 128
high potassium/low sodium, 105, *122*
omega fats and, 134
recommended, 130, 135, 173, *182*
satisfying effect, 131, 173

B

Bacon, 119, 173
 insulin index and, 154, 158
 liver stress and, 101, 104, 135

Bananas, 117, *122*, 158, 160, 313

Basic eating plan, 3, 165–166, 171
 guidelines, 188–189
 quick small meals, *190*
 salad ideas, 191
 three-day menu sample, *189–190*
 what to expect, 192

Beans, 186, 205

Beets, 63, 104, 121, 141, 174

Belly fat, 21, 155, 229, 245
 cortisol and, 245
 as fuel, 138, 153, 206
 insulin-resistance symptom, 156

Berries, 117, 124, 178, 205

Beverages
 alcoholic, 90, 138–139, 144, 205
 apple cider vinegar & lemon, 187–188
 beer alternative, 306, *306*
 carbohydrate, 81
 Dr. Berg's Meal Replacement Shake,
  304, *304*
 green vegetables as basis for, 124
 kombucha tea, 189, 306, *306*, 316
 milkshake alternative, 304, *304*
 recommended, *215*
 shakes, 124
 soda alternatives, 305, *305*
 stevia-sweetened, *305*
 substitution chart, *213*
 sugary, 213
 water, chlorine in, 213
 wine, 90, 306, *306*
 See also Soda pop; Wine; *specific beverages*
  by name

Bile, 102, 111, 169–170

Bile salts (purified), 91, 111

Birch sugar. *See* Xylitol

Birth-control pills, 94, 140, 207, 315

Bladder issues, 52, 227

Bloating, 167, 176, 177
 bile salts and, 169
 cruciferous vegetables and, 124, 125,
  186, 221, 314
 fats and, 135, 138, 171, 198
 Liver type and, 97, 101, 104
 menstrual cycle, 71
 nuts and, 182, 184, 312, 313, 318
 protein and, 205
 sugar alcohols and, 144
 water causing, 61
 weight loss and, 167, 221, 225, 313

Blood, pH levels, 49–50

Blood pressure, 57, 102
 adrenal glands and, 56–57
 insulin and, 157
 insulin medications and, 163
 potassium-sodium relationship,
  105, 157
 Ragland's test, 57, *58*

Blood sugar, 62, 117, 162

Blood sugar levels, 62–63, *63*, *117*, 131
 diabetes and, 204
 hypoglycemia, 204–205

Blood vessels, adrenal hormones and, 56–57

Body pH. *See* pH

Body temperature, 80

Body types, 3, 196
 characteristics, *8*, *9*, 10
 eating plans for, 165, 195
 enhancing results, 193, 196
 exercise and, 20
 glandular problems and, 9–10
 hormones and, 8–10
 mixed type, 41, 196
 quiz, 37–41
 See also Adrenal body type; Liver body
  type; Ovary body type; Thyroid
  body type

Boredom, eating out of, 136, 221

Brain fog, 54, *55*, 62, 133

Breads, 104, 130, 177, 205, 213, 315
    cravings for, 3, 15, 80, *81*
    empty nutrition, 191
    gluten and, 170
    glycemic index and, 153
    refined carbohydrates/grains, 81, 103,
        105, 197
    sugars in, 116–117, 172
    whole-wheat, 213, 320

Breakfast, 166, 172–173
    skipping, 152, 313

Broccoli, *122*, 125, 174
    bloating and, 186, 313
    cancer prevention, 13, 93
    constipation and, 224
    liver health and, 199
    sensitivity to, 177, 312

Broccoli sprouts, 176, 318

Brussels sprouts, 91, *122*, 125, 174, 206
    bloating and, 313
    cancer prevention, 13, 93

Burping, 19, 101, 104, 108, 169, 198

Butter, *212*, 319
    grass-fed, 176, *182*, 201
    recommended, 135, 158, 198

C

Cabbage, 13, *122*, 125, 174

Caffeine, 139–140, 207

Calcium, 24, 50, 140
    adrenal hormones and, 49, 50
    deficiency, 63
    deposits, 121
    loss of, 50
    sleep and, 50
    sources, 50
    supplements, 111

Calories, 248, 314–315
    exercise effects, 248

    fat-burning hormones and, 10–11
    hormones and, 249
    nutritional deficiencies and, 89

Cancer, 13, 30, 74, 111
    anti-cancer foods, 13, 93, 125
    beef and, 134, 317
    omega-3 fatty acids and, 134
    rBST and, 200
    sulforaphane and, 199

Candida, 104, 141

Carbohydrates, 153
    at bedtime, 110
    beverages, 81
    changed into fat, 130
    cravings for, 80, 81, *81*
    defined, 80–81
    fat-burning inhibited by, 48, 82
    fat-making-hormone triggers, 11
    function, 130
    hidden, 110
    liver stress, 199
    refined, 81, 82, 103, 120, 162, 191
    sweet, 20, 81
    thyroid function and, 77
    weight gain and, 130

Carcinogens, endocrine disrupters as, 30

Cataracts, kale effects on, 175

Cauliflower, 31, *122*, 125, 174, 177

Celery, 121, *122*, 125, 174
    before bed, 111, 148, 316
    dips for, 184, 186, *190*

Cellulite, 10, 246, 267, 315

Cereals, 177, 205
    craving, for energy, 15
    liver stress and, 104
    oatmeal, 170
    puffed, 116, 320
    refined, 81, 105, 116, 197

Cheese, 173, 176, 321
    Brie, amino acids in, 128
    calcium source, 50
    cravings for, 60, *60*, 63, 64

growth hormones and, 141, 201
live enzymes in, 128
protein source, *216, 217*
recommended, 135, 173, 176, *182*
satisfying effect, 131, 158, 173
whole-milk, 127
See also Dairy products

Chicken. *See* Poultry

Chlorophyll, 168, 170

Chocolate, 81, 117
alternatives, *211,* 307, *307*
caffeine in, 54, 139, 140
cravings for, 3, 60, 62
stimulant, 59

Cholesterol, 82, 118, 130, 218, 314
carbohydrate conversion into, 82,
     104, 130
drugs, 104, 140
eggs and, 107–108, 130, 181, 215,
     216–218, 313
enzyme effect on, 142
fatty foods and, 108, 130, 135
high levels explained, 82, 119, 130
insulin and, 35, 110, 150
lecithin antidote to, 130, 135, 181, 217
liver and, 107
pecans and, 183
thyroid influence on, 77

Choline, 199, 216

Circadian rhythm, 50–51, *51*

Cleanses, juice, 322

Coconut flour, 306

Coffee, 32, 166, 188–189
Adrenal types and, 54, 59, 139
decaffeinated, 139, *212,* 323
green tea vs., 55
liver stress and, 139

Cognitive function. *See* Memory

Collagen, 33, 108, 128
stomach acid and, 129

Constipation, 168–169, 224, 312
beets and, 104, 141

digestive issue, 167
Liver type and, 101, 103
weight loss and, 167, 225

Corn, 80, 117, 173, 176, 205
See also Genetically modified foods

Cortisol, 35, 139, 155, 229
Adrenal body type and, 47, 188, 245
alcohol trigger, 139
beets and, 141
belly fat and, 245
body-protein destruction, 47, 108, 128
caffeine and, 139
circadian rhythms and, 50–52, *51*
cutting calories and, 315
exercise and, 146–147, 160, 245, 261
growth-hormone inhibition, 109,
     110, 139
insulin medications and, 163
muscle breakdown and, 46, 47, 109, 146
pain and, 146, 317
sleep and, 146, 148, 162, 317
stress and, 12, 47, 146, 157, 162
test, 44

Cosmetics, chemicals in, 142

Crackers, 81, 104, 116, 172, 177

Cramps
in calf muscles, 50
menstrual cycle, 71, *71*
pH imbalance and, 188

Cravings. *See* Food cravings

Cruciferous vegetables, 31, 125, 175, 177
benefits, 125
cancer prevention, 13, 93
constipation and, 169, 224
for detoxification, 13, 141
iodine and, 91, 175, 202
named, 13, 125, 199
properties, 93
See also Vegetables; *specific vegetables
     by name*

Cysts, 13, 73, 89, 201, 315
See also Polycystic ovarian syndrome

D

Dairy products
estrogen in, 90
grass-fed/organic, 90, 166, 176, 320
hormones in, 27, 141, 200–201
milk, *122*, 176, 210, *215*
pasteurized, 50, 127, *212*
pesticides in, 28
See also Cheese

Dates, 117, 205

DDT (pesticide), 29–30, *29*, 141
liver and, 104
ovaries and, 72
thyroid and, 90

Dehydration, 60, 121, 144, 188

DES. *See* Diethylstilbestrol

Detoxification
foods needed for, 141
liver's role in, 140–141

Diabetes, 137, 155, 227
body proteins and, 129
hypoglycemia and, 204
insulin and, 35, 127, 132, 150
pork for diabetics, 180
potassium and, 162
sleep and, 162
unhealthy body and, 12
vitamin B$_1$ and, 162

Diet
anti-temptation cards, *220*
discouragement from no results,
220–221
eating habits, 118, 136, 221
sticking to a, 1, 21, 219–224
stress eating, 219–220
temptation, 219

Diethlystilbestrol (DES), 29

Diets, 5, 7–8
compared, 115–116, 130
everything in moderation, 20, 116, 145
high-fat, 115
high-protein, 258
low-calorie, 89, 115
low-fat, 115, 130
See also Eating habits

Digest Formula, 167, 169, 204

Digestive weaknesses, 167

Dining. *See* Eating out

Dinner foods, 166, 174

Dips, 184, 186, *190*, *214*

Dr. Berg's blog, 7

Dr. Berg's Body Type Program, 3–4
educational step, 1
goal, 23, 165, 320, 323
healing indicators, 19, 192, 195, 204,
225, 309
lifestyle change, 3
what to expect, 17–18, 192

Dr. Berg's Exclusive Membership site, 5, 354

Dr. Berg's YouTube channel, 223, 317, 354

Drinks. *See* Beverages

Drugs. *See* Medications

Dulse, 175

E

Ears, ringing in, 57

Eating habits
boredom and, 136, 221
clean-plate indoctrination, 222
craving sweets, 118, 221
discouragement with diet, 220–221
food as self-reward, 222
good intentions and, 118
social situations, 222–223
stress eating, 219–220
See also Foods

Eating out, 222–223

Eating plan, 165

Edema, 102, 105

Eggs, 131, 173, 176, 181, 314

benefits, 216–218, *217*
cholesterol and, 107–108, 130, 313–314
hard-boiled, 128
insulin response, 153, 154
omelets, 218, *218*
pasture-raised/organic, 134, 173, 181, 201, *212*
protein source, 173, 179, *217*, *218*
sulfur in, 93
whites, 153, 154
yolks, 127, 153, 154, 217–218, 314

Endocrine disruptors, 16, 27–29, 141, 207
as carcinogens, 30
DDT, 29, *29*, 141
hormones and, 28–29, *28*, 141

Endocrine system, 23–24
gland blockers and, 212
weight problem and, 115, 121, 312

Energy, fat as potential, 2, 14–15, 131, 267–268

Energy systems, 250
aerobic, 250–252, *251*, *252*
anaerobic, 252–253, *253*

Environmental chemicals
hormones and, 16, 24, 27–30, 72, 88
liver function, 102, 140–141

Enzyme inhibitors, 184–185, 312, 318

Enzymes, 6, 142
lipases, 135, 142
pancreas and, 142, 169
stomach acid and, 168

EPA. *See* U.S. Environmental Protection Agency

Epinephrine. *See* Adrenaline

Epstein-Barr virus (EVB), 88

Erythritol, 118, 144, 171, 205, *211*, *214*, 307, 319

Essential nutrients, 6–7
in eggs, 216

Estrogen, 13, 35, 70–71, 140
adrenal gland blockage from, 207

in animal feed, 90
beets and, 141
diethlystilbestrol (DES), 29
effects from meats, 90
exposure, symptom delays, 90
gland-blocking effect, 207
in milk, 90
in Ovary body type, 70–73
pregnancy and, 202
red wine and, 90
synthetic, 93–94
thyroid function and, 73, 89–90, 202, 203
triggers in foods, 89
See also Hormones

Exercise, 145–146, 159–160
Adrenal body type and, 20, 21, 53, 55, 159, 198, 245, 247, 257
body types and, 20
calorie burning by, 145, 248
cortisol and, 146
difficulty level, 255, *260*, 261
duration, 208, 256, *264*
eating and, 249
fat-burning effects, 145–146, 246, 248, 252, *264*, 266
fatigue and, 246, 268
frequency, 256
growth hormone and, 110
hormones and, 247–248, 255, 257, 258–259, *259*
insulin resistance effect, 159–160
intensity, 255, 257, 263, 316
metabolism speed-up, 316
muscle mass and, 248
Pilates, 159, 198
pulse rate, 256
quitting too soon, 266
resting between, 249, 257
sore muscles and, 249
soreness from, 261
stress effects, 146–147
sugar effects on, 119, 148
switching types of, 257

to trigger fat-burning, 21
types of, 256–257
walking, 57, 189, 198, 252, 267
weight loss and, 21, 145, 158, 248, 316
weight plateaus and, 257
weight training, 147, 253, 256, 257,
260, 264
where to start, 248
See also Aerobic exercise;
Anaerobic exercise
Eyebrow loss, 79, *79*
Eyelids
itchy and swollen, 99
sagging, 86
Eyes, puffiness around, 86

F

Facial hair, 49, *49*
Fasting
insulin and, 137, *137*, 151, 156
intermittent, 89, 136–138, 152–154,
158, 171, 206
Fat
defined, 2, 14–15
dietary, 207
in egg yolks, 217
as fuel source, 8–9, 18, *18*, 131
insulin and, *129*, 139, 180
liver stress and, 129
loss, 4, 21, 149, 192, 309
muscle mass and, 248
as potential energy, 2, *2*, 14–15, *15*,
131, 267–268
sugar and, 131
as survival mechanism, 12, 17, 18,
23, 149
Fat burning
all foods in moderation, 20, 116, 145
healing phase, *18*
insulin and, 120, *120*, 144, 158
protein and, 128
sleep and, 19, 20, 147–148, 208,
249, 317
snacking effects on, 158–159
sugar effect on, 9, 18
triggers and blockers, 9, 19–20
Fat-burning hormones, 2, 10–11, 13,
15, 33–34
calories and, 10–11
cortisol and, 254
exercise and, 145–146, 246–248,
252, 253, 255, 258, *259*
fats and, 315
insulin and, 48, 120
liver and, 26, 94, 106, 175, 258
nullification of, 15, 19, 115, 120,
148, 249
pain effect on, 53
potassium and, 115
protein and, 126
sleep and, 52, 110, 249
sugar and, 47, 48, 118, 119, 148
weight loss and, 20
See also Hormones
Fat-burning triggers, 115
exercise, 145–146
fats, 129–135
gland destroyers, 138–142
protein, 126–129
skipping meals & fasting, 136–138
sleep, 147–148
stress, 146–147
sugar absence, 116–120
vegetables, 121–125
water retainers, 143–144
Fatigue, 223, 226
Adrenal body type and, 53–54, *53*
exercise and, 246
reasons for, 226, 314
thyroid gland and, 79
See also Sleep
Fat-making hormones. *See* Fat-storing
hormones

Fats, 11, 129–130
 adding to meals, 126, 138, 158
 amounts to eat, 181–182, *182*, 207
 to avoid, 182, 207, *212*
 bile and, 102, 111, 167, 169, 198
 body's use of, 130
 butter, 158, 201
 coconut oil, 135, 198, 203
 dangers of, 315
 dietary, 130, 154, 207
 essential, 133–134
 as fuel source, 8–9, 131
 hunger and, 158, 207
 hydrogenated, 134, *212*, 315
 insulin and, *129*, 138, 154, 158
 liver and, 93, 102, 104
 as obesity cause, 129
 omega-3, 133–134
 omega-6, 134
 recommended, 135, *182*
 saturated, 135, 198
 sugar and, 8, 18, 104
 trans fats, 134–135, 182

Fat-storing hormones, 15, 19–20, 35
 dietary fat and, 129, 314
 effect of cortisol, 35, 250
 exercise and, 145
 fat-burner nullification, 115
 foods to counteract, 31
 insulin, 48, 116
 sugar and, 48, 116
 triggers, 11, 19–20, 315
 See also Hormones

Fatty acids, 6, 128, 133–134

Feet, cold, 80, *80*

Fiber, 169, 199, 224, 312

Fibromyalgia, 52–53, 229

Figs, 117, 205

Fingernails, 84, 85
 amino-acid building blocks, 6
 body proteins and, 84, 85, 128–129
 brittle, 13, 85
 enzymes and, 142

 hormones and, 4, 258
 ridges on, 85, *85*
 thyroid and, 77, 84

Fish, 179, 180, 181
 to avoid, 180
 farm-raised, 72, 128, 134, *212*, 317
 healthiest, 180
 hormones in, 72, 90, 141, 201
 meats vs., 32, 106
 mercury in, 141, 215
 tuna, 141, 180
 wild-caught, 180, 201, 317
 See also Seafood

Flour alternatives, 306

Fluid retention. *See* Water retention

Fluids. *See* Beverages; Liquids; Water;
 specific fluids by name

Food
 defined, 5–6
 as self-reward, 222
 temptations, 219

Food cravings, 60, 63, 131, 138
 adrenal deficiency and, 62
 for carbs, 80, 228
 concentrated nutrition and, 3, 191
 decrease in, 18, 19, 167, 195
 fats and, 158, 207
 fatty foods, 104
 insulin resistance and, 156, 204, 228
 licorice, 63, 319
 Liver type and, 101, *101*
 low-calorie diets and, 89
 between meals, 206
 Ovary type and, 71
 salty foods, 60, *60*, 319
 sweets, 62, 133, 156, 221, 228
 Thyroid type and, 80, *81*
 See also Hunger

Food labels, 31, 32, 201
 reading, importance of, 110, 144,
  158, 319
 for vitamins, 105, 311

Foods
    addictive chemicals in, 210
    cage-free, 201
    fermented, 104, 159
    free-range, 134, 201, *212*
    gas-producing, 184, 312–313
    for healing, 6, 13, 121
    high-potassium, 105, *122*, 160–161, 309
    hormone-free, 141, 201, 311
    natural, 32, 209–210
    non-foods vs., 6–7
    organic, 32, 128, 180–181, 201, 210, *212*
    pasture-raised, 134, 180–181, 201
    pleasure foods, 166–167, 222, 283–303
    protein amounts in, 216, *216–217*
    refined, 80–81, 103–104, 105,
        116–117, 215
    water-retaining (chart), *214*
    See also Eating habits; Genetically
        modified foods; *specific foods by
        type or name*
Food sensitivities, 177, 312–313
    dairy products, 176
    eggs, 173, 216
    grains, 117
    Liver type and, 97
    nuts, 182
    salt, 157
    See also Allergies
Forks over Knives (film), 179
Fructose, 118, 171
Fruit juices, 103
    orange juice, 116, 148
Fruits, 205
    acceptable (list), 178
    canned, 117, 205
    dried, 117, 205
    hormone health and, 205
    nutrients in, 178
    off-limits (list), 178
    potassium in, *122*, 208
    sugar in, 117, 177–178
    See also Berries; *specific fruits by name*

Fungicides. *See* Pesticides
Future of Food (video), 321, 355

G

Gallbladder, 87, 91, 169–170
    acupressure for, 199
    bile and, 91, 111, 167
    caffeine and, 139
    fats and, 129, 135, 138, 196
    inflammation effects, 229
    nuts and, 183
    symptoms, 107–108
    thyroid deficiencies, 202–203
Gallbladder Formula
    bile deficiency, 111, 167, 169
    bloating, 167
    digestive issues, 167
    fat digestion, 138
    fibromyalgia on right side, 229
    missing/sluggish gallbladder, 91,
        111, 180
    peanut butter consumption, 127
    thyroid support, 203
Garlic, 93, 142, 174
Genetically modified foods (GMOs),
        30–31, 201, 321
GERD. *See* Acid reflux
GH. *See* Growth hormone
Gland blockers, 207
    substitutes (chart), *212*
Gland destroyers, 138–139, 138–142
Glands, 24–26
    body types and, 9
    hormones and, 25–26, *25*
    interaction of, 86–87
    problem causes, 26–30
Glucagon, 34, 118
    exercise and, 145, 247, 258, *259*
    protein and, 119, 126, 204
Glutamine, 170

Gluten, 100, 101, 170

Glycemic index, 153

Glycerol, 205

Glycine, 128, 314

Glyphosate, 30, 201

GMOs. *See* Genetically modified foods

Grains, 101, 177
    alternative flours, 306
    hormone health and, 205
    refined vs. whole, 116–117
    sugar and, 116, 177

Graves' disease, 87, 202

Green tea, 55, 140, *212, 215*

Growth hormone (GH), 13, 33,
        109–111, 119
    adrenal hormones and, 41
    cortisol increase and, 139
    estrogen and, 125
    exercise and, 110, 145, 146, 254, 255
    fat-burning effects during sleep, 147, 148
    fuel regulation and, 110
    insulin-like growth factor (IGF)
        triggered by, 33, 127
    protein and, 119, 126
    side effects, 111
    sugar and, 110, 119
    See also Hormones

Growth hormones, 141
    agricultural use, 27, 32, 72, 209
    in foods, 24, 141, 210, 267, 315
    liver damage and, 93–94
    Thyroid body type and, 90

Guyton, Arthur C., 136, 151

H

Hair, thyroid effects on, 79, 84
    See also Facial hair

Hashimoto's disease, 87, 202

Head injury, fatigue and, 226, *226*

Health & Wellness Center, 5

Health & Wellness Center products,
    351–353

Health, defined, 149

Health factors, 195

Heavy metals
    detoxification of, 140
    endocrine disruptors, 28, 141

Herbal stimulants, 66, 139

Herbicides, 27, 30, 32, 107, 207
    See also Pesticides

High-fructose corn syrup, 116, 177, *214*

Honey, 118, *122*, 171, 205

Hormone health
    eating rules, 205–208
    sleep and, 208
    starches and, 205

Hormone replacement therapy (HRT),
    72, 74, 93–94, 310

Hormones, 23–24, 119
    age and, 23
    anaerobic exercise and, 258–259, *259*
    anti-fat-making-hormone foods, 31–32
    body shapes and, 8–10, 23
    calories and, 249
    defined, 2, 24–25
    endocrine disruptors and, 28–29
    environmental, 16, 24, 72
    estrogen, 34, 35, 89
    exercise and, 247–248, 258, *259*
    fat and, 17–18, 129
    fat-making, 2, 11, 110, 129, 144, 210
    fat-storing, 15, 19–20, 35
    in food, 27, 141, 315
    glands and, 25–26, *25*
    glucagon, 34, 118
    insulin-like growth factor (IGF), 33, 127
    liver damage and, 127
    in meat products, 16, 141
    in milk, 200, 201
    miscommunication methods,
        28–29, *28*

pesticides and, 29, *29*
protein and, 204
rBST, 200, 201
sleep and, 4, 24, 50–52, *51*
sugar and, 119
testosterone, 34, 49
thyroid, 34
weight loss and, 2, 12
See also Adrenaline; Cortisol; Fat-
    burning hormones; Fat-storing
    hormones; Growth hormone;
    Insulin; Thyroid hormones

Hot flashes, 74, *74*, 227, 230

HRT. *See* Hormone replacement therapy

Hummus, 181, 186, 205

Hunger
    fats and, 158, 207
    between meals, 206
    See also Food cravings

Hydrocortisone. *See* Cortisol

Hydrogenated oils, 134–135, 142, 184, *212*

Hypercholesterolemia, 82

Hypoglycemia, 204
    diabetes and, 204
    memory problems and, 227
    protein and, 204–205

I

Immune system, adrenal hormones and,
    44, 63

Indigestion, 129, 168

Infections, thyroid function and, 88

Inflammation, 229
    adrenal hormones and, 52–53, *52*,
        63–64
    enzymes and, 142
    grain products and, 100, 170
    reduction of, 195, 225
    stress and, 146, 250
    weight loss and, 225, 248

Insecticides. *See* Pesticides

Insulin, 35, 132, *132, 133*, 136, 150–151
    alcoholic beverages and, 138–139
    apple cider vinegar and, 187
    fasting and, 137, *137*, 152
    fat and, *129*, 138, 154, 172, 180
    fat burning and, 118, 120, *120*, 144
    functions, 132
    growth hormone and, 110
    inflammation and, 229
    medication effects, 163
    memory problems and, 227
    polycystic ovarian syndrome and, 156
    potassium and, 160
    protein and, 119, 126, *126*
    snacking and, 126, 136, 152, 153, 206
    spike, causes (list), 157
    stress and, 146
    sugar and, 48, 119, 129, *129*, 150
    triggers, 136, *136*, 138, 151, 153–154

Insulin index, 153, 154–155

Insulin-like growth factor (IGF),
    33, *112*, 127

Insulin resistance, 131–132, *132*,
    155–156, *156*
    blood pressure and, 157
    corrective actions, 158–159
    fermented foods for, 159
    food cravings, 206, 228
    improvement signs, 204
    symptoms of (list), 156
    urination and, 227

Intermittent fasting. *See* Fasting

Iodine, 175, 186, 201
    cruciferous vegetables and, 91, 125, 202
    for Ovary body type, 201
    sea kelp, 91, 125, 175, 201

Iron deficiency, 63

Irritable bowel syndrome (IBS), 170

Isolated food factors, 6

Itching, 63, 99, 102, 314

J

Juice cleanses, 322
Juices, fruit, 103, 116, 213
Juicing, of vegetables, 124, 206, 322

K

Kale, 125, 174, 175
    bloating and, 221, 314
    constipation and, 169, 224, 312
    high potassium/low sodium, *122*
    oxalates in, 186, 321–322
Kale shakes, 124, 171, 175, 178, 208
Kefir, 128, 201, *211*, 321
Kelp. *See* Sea kelp
Ketchup, 116, 172, *214*, 319
Ketosis, 165–166, 223
Kettle Chips, 144
Kidney stones, 121, 321–322
    lemon juice and, 159, 187

L

Lecithin, 130, 135, 181, 217, 313
Lee, John, 88
Legs, calf-muscle cramps, 50
Legumes, 186
Lemons, 178, 187, 205, *211*
Lentils, 181, 186, 188, 205
Licorice, cravings for, 63, 319
Liquids, 171
    frequency of use, *215*
    recommended (chart), *215*
    See also Beverages; Water
Liver, 93, *94*
    alcohol and, 95–96, 138–139
    bile, 102, 198
    caffeine and, 139–140
    cirrhosis, 102–103, 139
    coffee and, 139
    damage, testing for, 105–106
    detoxification by, 140–141
    fat-burning hormones and, 26, 94,
        106, 175, 258
    fats and, 104, 115, 129, 135, 198
    foods for healing, 93, 95, 106, 199
    functions, 93, 102, 140–141
    itching and, 99, 102, 314
    malfunctioning, 93–96, 102–103
    nutrients for, 199
    problem causes, 26–30, 93–94,
        104–105
    protein intake, 126, 127, 198, 312
    skin appearance and, 102, 142
    stressors, 103–104, 106, 135, 140,
        181, 199
    sugar and, 103
    thyroid hormones and, 14
    toxic chemicals and, 104
Liver body type, *8, 9,* 10, 94–95, *95, 96, 97*
    abdominal fluid, 94–96, *96*
    acupressure technique for,
        199–200, *200*
    carbohydrates for, 199
    causes, 103–105
    characteristics, 44, 97–103, *97,*
        111–113, *112*
    eating plan, 198–199
    exercise for, 246, 253
    fats for, 129, 198
    food cravings, 101
    minerals for, 199
    personality, 99
    proteins for, 106, 127, 198
    symptoms, 99–100, 102–103, 113–114
    vegetables for, 93, 95, 106, 199
Liver spots, 102, 108–109, *112*
Lotions, skin absorption of, 142
Lunch foods, 166, 173–174

M

Mangoes, 117

Mannitol, 144

Maple syrup, 307
  Joseph's Sugar-Free Maple Syrup, 307

Massage tool, 231, *231*, 232, *232*, *233*
  adrenal points, 243–244, *243*, *244*
  collarbone points, 241–242, *242*
  lower-neck points, 238–239, *238*
  mid-back points, 239–241, *240*, *241*
  mid-neck points, 237, *237*
  occipital points, 235–236, *235*, *236*
  rules for use, 232
  stress points, *233*, 234
  upper-neck points, 234–235, *234*, *235*
  See also Acupressure

Meals
  breakfast, 152, 166, 172–173, 313
  dinner, 174
  lunch, 173–174
  number per day, 206
  overview, 166, 171
  skipping, 136–138, 152–153, 166

Meats, 16, 104, 106
  beef, *122*, 317
  best types, 207, *212*
  fish vs., 32, 108
  grass-fed/organic, 128, 134, 180, 201
  hormones in, 16, 90, 141
  pesticide residues in, 28, 32
  pork, 180
  processed, 119, 180, 207
  sugars in, 119
  trimming fat from, 32
  See also Poultry

Medications, 163, 310
  cortisol synthetics, 229
  Coumadin, 310
  gland blocking, 207
  insulin and, 163
  psychiatric, 140, 163
  side effects, 104, 140, 155

thyroid, 89, 175, 230
  See also specific medications by name

Melons, 63, 117, 178

Memory, 102, 156, 227

Menopause, 73–74, 88
  body type change and, 74
  hot flashes, 73, 74, *74*, 227, 230
  Ovary type symptoms (list), 75

Menstrual cycle, 71, 79, 230

Mercury, 141, 215

Metabolism, 78
  body temperature and, 80
  dieting and, 149–150
  thyroid gland and, 80

Milk, 176
  estrogen in, 90
  hormones in, 27, 141, 200–201
  pasteurized, 50, 127, *212*

Minerals
  adrenal function and, 44
  depletion from stimulants, 66
  diuretics and, 140
  in eggs, 216
  germination effect, 185
  health factor, 6
  kombucha tea and, 306
  for liver, 199
  protein formation and, 129
  in sea kelp, 125, 203
  in sea salt, 60
  for thyroid, 203
  in vegetables, 121, 199, 206
  water flushing out, 62
  See also Calcium; Potassium

Monosodium glutamate (MSG), 105,
     172, 206, 318
  insulin effects, 144, 207
  water retention from, 143, 207, *214*

Monsanto Company, 30–31

Muscle mass, fat-burning and, 248

Muscle proteins, as fuel instead of fat, 17, 46

Muscles. *See* Exercise

Mushrooms, 108, *122*, 128, 175, 181

Myxedema, 10, 83

N

Nails. *See* Fingernails

Natural foods, 32, 209–210

Neck points, 204, 234–235, 237–239

Night-time eating, 110, 118, 136, 174

Nutrients, essential, 6–7

Nutritional supplements. *See* Supplements

Nuts, 129, 130, 173, 180, 182–183
    almonds, 128, 134, 182, 318
    amino acids in, 128
    amounts to eat, 134, 135, 181–182
    benefits, 131
    bloating and, 135, 182, 184, 312, 313
    cashews, 313, 318
    eating too many, 183–184
    enzyme inhibitors and, 184–185,
        312, 318
    enzymes and, 142
    gallbladder and, 183
    germinating, 185, 312, 318
    iodine and, 175
    omega fatty acids in, 133, 134
    pecans, 128, 182, 183
    pistachios, 183
    recommended (list), 182–183
    roasted, 127, 184, 185, 318
    storing, 183
    walnuts, *122*, 128, 133, 134, 182,
        183, 318

O

Obesity
    America vs. other countries, 26–27
    fats and, 129

    healthiness and, 12–15
    liver and, 103

Oils, 130, 177, 182, 198

Olives, 175, *182*
    cholesterol-free, 130
    omega-6 fat in, 134
    recommended, 158, 173

Omega fatty acids, 128, 133–134, 317

Onions, 93, 142, 175

Organic Cruciferous Superfood, 91, 186

Organic, defined, 32, 200

Organic foods, 141, 210

Osteoporosis, 24, 47, 50

Ovaries, 69, *69*, 72
    brain control of, 73
    menopause and, 73–74

Ovary body type, *8*, *9*, 10, 69–75
    causes, 72–73
    cellulite problems, 315
    characteristics, 44, 70, *70*
    cysts, 13, 73, 89, 201, 315
    eating plan, 73, 200–202
    estrogen and, 70, 71, 72–73
    exercise for, 246
    exercise plan, 267–268
    fats, 201
    iodine for, 201
    menstrual cycle and, 71
    nutrients for, 201–202
    pain in, 71
    phytonutrients for, 202
    proteins and, 127, 200
    stages of, 71, *72*
    symptoms (list), 75
    thyroid blockage, 73

Overeating, 103
    animal proteins, 181
    nuts, 183

Oxalates, 321–322

Oxygen, adrenal glands' effect on,
    55, 56–57

P

Pain
  effect on weight loss, 146, 248, 317
  gallbladder and, 107, 138, 183, 202, 229
  Ovary type and, 71
  pH imbalance symptom, 188
  in right shoulder, 98, *98*, 104, 138, 169
Pancreas
  enzymes and, 142
  nuts and, 184–185
Pasta, 177, 205
  cravings for, 81
  sugars in, 116, 172
Peanut butter, 127, 158, 183, 184
  amounts to eat, 182, *182, 216, 217*
Pesticides, 24, 27, 28, 209
  bodily storage of, 29, *29*
  DDT, 29–30, *29*, 141
  endocrine disruptors, 141, 207
  estrogen-like effects, 73
  in imported foods, 29–30
  mimicking of hormones, 16, 24, 90
  See also Herbicides
pH
  adrenals and, 49–50, 188, 197
  bodily levels (list), 187
  imbalance, symptoms of (list), 188
Pickles, 169, 319
Plastics, 28
Poisons, environmental, 27, 88
Polycystic ovarian syndrome (PCOS),
      89, 156, 157
Popcorn, 60, 319
Pork, 180, *212*
Potassium, 105, 115, 160–161
  adrenals and, 44, 49–50, 196–197
  body relaxation and, 118
  daily requirement, 123, 160,
      173–174, 206
  deficiency and high blood pressure, 157

depletion factors, 144
  fluid retention and, 121, 123, *123*
  foods high in, 121
      listed, *122*
  insulin and, 123, 157
  pills, 161
  in salads, 161, 206
  salt and, 208
  sodium and, 105, 143–144, 208
  sodium-potassium ratio, 121, 123, 309
  sugars and, 118, 144
  in vegetables, 121, *122*, 123, 141,
      143, 206
Potatoes, *122*, 144, 171, 176, 205
  conversion to fat, 80, 117
  sugars in, 172
Potbelly, 95–97, *95, 96, 97*, 106
Poultry, 180, *212*
  amino acids in, 128
  estrogen in feed for, 27, 90
  GMO feed, 180
  grown with hormones, 16, 27, 90
  nitrates in, 180
  omega fats in free-range, 134
  organic/pasture-raised, 180
  protein amounts, 179, *216, 217*
  skin on, 127
  trimming skin from, 32
  See also Meats
Prednisone, 63–64, 65, 140, 155, 229
Pregnancy, 310
  thyroid weakness and, 73, 86, 89,
      202, 230
Premenstrual syndrome (PMS), 71
Protein, 47, 126–129, 215–216
  amounts in foods, 215, *216*, 217, *217*
  amounts to eat, 207
  animal, 128, 179–180, 181
  in beans, 186
  blood-sugar levels and, 204
  body types and, 126, 127
  collagen, 128
  deficiency symptoms, 128

eating before exercise, 145
eating glucose with, 151
fat-burning hormones and, 125
forms of, 127
hormones and, 204
hypoglycemia and, 204–205
insulin and, 119, 126, 151, 153
as insulin trigger, 151, 153
liver and, 126, 312
meats, 207
soy, 6, 181, 207
sugar and, 47, 154, 204
symptom improvement signs, 205
thyroid functioning and, 84
vegetarian, 198
vegetarian (list), 181, *216*
whole, recommended, 127, 173

Protein isolates, 209
    MSG and, 143
    soy, 186, 207

Protein powder, 126, 127, 181

Protein shakes, 6, 173

Pthalides, 148, 316

R

Radiation, thyroid function and, 88

Raisins, 117, 205

Raw Wheat Grass Juice Powder, 168, 170

Recipes
    Almond Coconut Chocolates,
        293–294, *293, 294*
    Apple-cider vinegar & lemon drink, 187
    Asparagus and Tomato Frittata, 271
    Cauliflower Hot Wings, 284, *284*
    Cauliflower Mashed, 285, *285*
    Cauliflower Rice, 286, *286*
    Chicken Paprikash, 279
    Chicken with Asparagus, 278
    Chicken with Herbed Cheese, 281
    Comfort Cookies, 296, *296*
    Curried Chicken Salad, 274

    Curry Mayonnaise, 275
    Easy Meatloaf, 282
    Garlic Walnut Chicken, 277
    Guilt-Free Cookies, 291–292,
        291–292
    Healthy Pancakes, 290, *290*
    Healthy Peanut Butter Cups, 299, *299*
    Kale shakes, 124, 175
    Kale Slaw, 273
    Keto Bombs, 300, *300*
    Legal Brownies, 283, *283*
    Low-Carbohydrate Cheesecake,
        302–303, *303*
    No-Flour Amazing Pizza, 287–288, *287*
        parchment paper trick, 288
        toppings for, 287, *287*
    No-Grain English Muffins, 295, *295*
    No-Grain Granola, 297–298, *297*
    No-Sugar Chocolate Ice Cream, 301, *301*
    omelets, 218, *218*
    Sesame Ginger Kale Slaw, 272
    shakes, 124
    Spaghetti Squash with Tahini, 269
    Sugar Snap Peas with Lemon Mustard
        Dressing, 270
    Walnut Chicken, 276
    Warm Chicken Salad, 280
    Zucchini Pasta, 289, *289*

Restaurants
    eating at, 6, 189, 222–223
    MSG in food, 143, 172, 207

Rice, 101, 171, 177, 205

Rice cakes, 81, 116, 177, 320

Ritalin, 83

Russia, obesity in, 16

S

Saccharin. *See* Sugar substitutes

Salad dressings, 177, *214*
    MSG avoidance, 206
    sugar hidden in, 116, 172, 319

Salads, 124, 206
ideas for, 177,191
for lunch, 173
potassium source, 123, 161, *161*, 197

Salt, 60, 318
cravings for, 60, *60*, 319
potassium and, 105, 157, 208
sea salt vs. table salt, 60, 318, 319
See also Sodium

Sauerkraut, 104, 159, 169, 175

Seafood, 180
amino acids in, 128
for Thyroid type, 203
wild-caught, 201
See also Fish

Sea kelp, 91, 125, 175, 201

Seeds. *See* Nuts

Selenium, 125, 199

Serotonin, chocolate and, 62

Shomon, Mary, 88

Skin
absorption of cosmetics, 142
acne, 49, 157
cortisol and, 228
essential fatty acids and, 134
fat-soluble vitamins and, 91, 170
liver and, 100, 102, 142, 258
liver spots, 102, 108–109
sagging, 84, *85*, 128
thyroid functioning and, 77, 79, 84

Sleep, 110–111, 147–148, 162, 192, 227
acupressure techniques for, 146, 162
Adrenal type, 50, *50*, 53–54, 98
apnea, 227
bedtime and, 316–317
bedtime eating effects, 148
calcium and, 50
circadian rhythms, 50–51, *51*, *147*
cortisol and, 51, 141, 148, 162, 317
cycles, 50, 51, 148
dreams, 148, 224
exercise and, 145, 159, 189, 208

fat burning and, 19, 52, 110, 147–148, 208, 249
growth hormone and, 109, 147, *147*, 317
healing indicator, 19, 149, 195, 221
hormones and, 4, 50–52, 147–148, *147*, 208
importance of, 208, 248, 249
insulin and, 162
interrupted, 148, 227
Liver type, 98–99
nutritional supplementation and, 148
protein amount and, 205, 207
recommendations for, 316
See also Fatigue

Snacks, 126, 158–159, 166, 171, 190
bedtime, 148, 316
insulin trigger, 126, 136, 152, 153, 206
substitute, *211*

Social eating, 222–223

Soda pop, 139–140
alternatives, 305, *305*
caffeine in, 54, 140
diet, 144
sugar in, 116

Sodium, 105, 144
dehydration and, 60
fluid retention and, 60, 118, 121, 123, 213
in MSG, 105, 207
potassium and, 105, 144, 208
sodium-potassium ratio, 121, 123, 309
sugar and, 118, 144
in vegetables, 121, *122*
See also Salt

Soft drinks. *See* Soda pop

Solvents, 28

Sore muscles, 52, 249

Soy, 173, 181, 267
GMO, 30, 31, 186
oil, 177, 182, 198
products, 89, 186, 321
protein isolate, 6, 143, 186, 207

Soybeans, 186

Speech, thyroid effects on, 86

Spices, 143, 177, 318

Splenda, 55

Sprouts, 176, 313, 318

Starches, 117, 144, 176, 205
  hormone health and, 205

Steroids, 65

Stevia, 118, 171, 205, *211*, *214*, 307, 319
  in beverages, 171, 187, 305, *305*
  flavored, 305, *305*
  in vegetable blends, 124, 175, 206

Stimulants, 59, 66
  herbal, 66, 139

Stomach acidity, 128–129, 168, 169

Stress, 146, 148, 220, 250
  acupressure for, 228, 231
  adrenal hormones and, 50, 58, 202,
    228, 247
  anti-stress activities, 147
  autoimmune conditions and, 202–203
  calming nutrients, 220
  cortisol increase from, 146, 250
  exercise benefit, 146, 250
  insulin and, 146
  releasing techniques, 198
  tolerance, 149, 228
  types of, 146

Stress eating, 219–220

Stress hormone. *See* Cortisol

Sugar, 110, 158, 171, 205, 210
  absence of, 116–119
  Adrenal type and, 48
  agave, 118, 171, 205
  aging effects, 119
  body storage of, 118
  in carrot juice, 179
  cravings for, 62, 206, 221, 228
  eating at bedtime, 148
  exercise and, 119, 148, 266
  fat and, 8, 131

fat-burning hormones and, 47
fat burning inhibited by, 82, 117–119,
  117, 266
foods that turn into, 116–117, 171, 177
fructose, 118
in fruits, 117, 177–178
as fuel source, 9, 18, 131
glycogen, 150, 160, 204
grains and, 177
hidden, 103, 116–117, 172, 188,
  210, 319
high-fructose corn syrup, 116, 177, *214*
honey, 118, 171, 205
hormones and, 110, 119
insulin and, 48, 116, 119, *120*,
  131–132, 150, 151, 157
Liver type and, 99, 103–104
potassium and, 118, 144
protein and, 47, 119, 154, 204
synthetic, 142
water retention and, 118
See also Blood sugar

Sugar substitutes, 118, 144, 171, *211*,
  214, 319
  agave, 118, 171, 205
  aspartame, 144, *214*
  erythritol, 118, 144, 171, 205, 307, 319
  hormone aggravation, 55
  isomalto-oligosaccharides (IMO), 307
  Maple Syrup, Joseph's Sugar-Free, 307
  Splenda, 55
  stevia, 118, 171, 205, 305, *305*, 307, 319
  sugar alcohols, 118, 144
  water retention and, 144
  xylitol, 118, 144, 166, 205, 307, 319

Supper. *See* Dinner foods

Supplements, 311
  acidifier, 168
  calcium, 111
  food vs., 121, 123, 128, 134
  Organic Cruciferous Superfood, 91, 186
  sleep and, 148
  thyroid weakness and, 82

Sweeteners. *See* Sugar; Sugar substitutes; *specific sweeteners by name*

Sweets, 219–220, 221, 228
blood sugar level and, 62, *63*
cell hunger and, 133
fat burning and, 20
insulin resistance and, 156, 204
liver stress from, 103
nutrient-dense foods and, 3
thirst from, 144

T

Taurine, 314

Tea, 139–140
green, 55, 140, *212, 215*
herbal, 140, 171, 188, *212, 213, 215*

Tempeh, 181, 186

Testosterone, 34, 49
anaerobic exercise and, 145, 254, 258, *259*
beets and, 141
low-fat diet and, 130
vitamin E and, 109

Textbook of Medical Physiology (Guyton), 136, 151

Thyroid body type, *8, 9,* 10, 77–92, *78, 83,* 202–203
acupressure technique for, 204
carbohydrate cravings, 80, *81*
causes, 88–89
eating plan, 203
estrogen avoidance, 90
exercise for, 246, 253
fats, 203
fluid weight, 10, 83
foods to avoid, 90
hair loss, 84, *84*
infections and, 88
nutrients for, 203
proteins and, 127, 203
stages, 83, *83*
symptoms (list), 92

Thyroid function, estrogen and, 89–90, 202

Thyroid gland, 77–78, *77*
attention deficit disorder (ADD) and, 83
body protein and, 84
body temperature and, 80
eye effects, 86
fatigue and, 79
iodine and, 91, 125, 175
liver function and, 14, 87, *87*
metabolism and, 78, 79
pesticides and, 90
secondary problem, 86–87, 89, 202
sluggishness symptoms, 79–82, 83
speech effects, 86
symptom-source questions, 88, 203
vitamin needs and, 82

Thyroid hormones, 14, 34, 202
deficiency, 88
environmental factors, 88
estrogen and, 13, 73, 87, 88, 89, 202
gallbladder and, 202
purpose, 78
pregnancy and, 89, 202
T3, 86, 125, 202
T4, 86–87, 125, 202
See also Hormones

Tinnitus (ringing in ears), 57

Tiredness. *See* Fatigue

Tofu, 181, 186

Tongue, indentations, 86, *86*

Trans fats, 134–135, 182

Tryptophan, 128

Turkey. *See* Poultry

Turmeric, 177

U

Ulcers, remedy for, 168

U.S. Environmental Protection Agency (EPA), 16, 27–28

V

Vaccines, 141

Valine, 128

Vegetable juice cleanse, 322

Vegetables, 103, 121–125, 312
  beverages from, 124
  bloating from, 176, 177
  cooked vs. raw, 121, 176
  cooking, 121, 176
  dislike of, 313
  fermented, 169
  iodine and, 91, 125
  leafy green, 50, 105, 108, 124, 206,
    321–322
  for Liver type, 95, 106
  nutrient-dense, 206
  as potassium source, 121, *122*, 123,
    141, 143, 206
  starchy, 117, 144, 176
  unlimited quantities (list), 174–175
  washing, 32
  See also Cruciferous vegetables; *specific
    vegetables by name*

Vegetable starches, 117

Vegetarianism
  drawbacks, 179
  gallbladder problems, 170
  hormone health and, 205
  proteins for (list), 181, 216

Vinegar. *See* Apple cider vinegar

Viruses, 63–64
  adrenals and, 65
  Epstein-Barr, 88
  filtered through liver, 93

Vitamins, 83, 104
  B vitamins, 105, 197, 311
    B₁, 162, 183
    caffeine effect on, 140
    in cruciferous vegetables, 199
    deficiency and dreaming, 224
    in eggs, 216

  fat burning and, 192, 223
  in nutritional yeast, 105, 162, 192,
    197, 223
  fat-soluble, 111, 169, 170, 179
  recommendations, 311
  synthetic, 6, 66, 105, 162, 311, 320
  thyroid weakness and, 82
  vitamin C, 65, 108, 196, 197, 318
  vitamin E, 108–109, 183

W

Water, 60, 188
  bloating from, 61
  carbonated, 188, *213*, *215*, 305
  chlorine in, *213*
  dehydration, 60, 121
  drinking large quantities, 61–62, 317
  sparkling, 140

Water retention, 115, 121, 143, 213
  alcohol and, 144
  artificial sweeteners and, 144
  food substitutes, *214*
  grains and, 116–117
  monosodium glutamate and, 143, 207
  potassium and, 123, *123*
  protein effect on, 315
  refined sugar and, 118, 144
  sodium and, 144, 207–208
  thyroid problem and, 83

Water weight, 4, 106, 143
  high-potassium foods and, 123, *123*
  losing, 4, 21, 192, 309
  sodium increase and, 144
  sodium-potassium imbalance, 115
  See also Weight loss

Websites, 351, 354

Weight, as symptom, 1–2, 13, 195, 225

Weight gain
  alcohol and, 138
  calories and, 10–11, 315
  carbohydrates vs. fat, 130
  cortisol and, 263

liver scarring and, 102–103
menopause and, 73
polycystic ovarian syndrome and,
    89, 157
thyroid function and, 10, 86
Weight goal, 4, 12, 17, 19, 195
Weight loss
    barriers (list), 248
    best indicators, 19, 192, 195,
        220–221, 225
    body conditions and, 225
    calorie-burning effects, 248
    educational step, importance of, 1
    healthiness and, 12–13
    hormone blockage and, 4
    hormones and, 2, 17
    maintaining, 3–4, 17–19
    muscle gain, 17, 192, 220
    plateaus, 156, 257
    problem identification and, 1–2
    sleep quality and, 192
    stress and, 310
    stubborn weight problem, 1–2
    sugar storage and, 18, *18*
    timeline for, *18*
    treatments for, 19
    water weight vs. fat, 115, 309
    weekly maximum fat loss, 4, 309
    See also Water weight
Weight-loss products, soy isolate in, 186
Weight plateaus, 156, 257
Wheat, 100
    See also Breads; Grains
Wheat germ, 108, 109
Willpower, 1, 222
Wine, 90, 130, 138–139, 205
    alternative to, 306, *306*
    effect on fat burning, 20, 110, 116, 148
    liver setback from, 96, 119, 138, 189, 323
    sugar hidden in, 116, 172, 188
    sulfites in, 140

X

Xylitol, 171, 307, 319
    acceptable sweetener, 118, 205, 307
    in coffee, 166, 189
    non-GMO, importance of, 118, 144
    sugar/sweetener substitute, *211*,
        214, 319

Y

Yeast, nutritional
    amount to take, 105, 162, 197
    B vitamins and, 105, 162, 192,
        197, 224
    how to take, 162, 223
    for nightmares, 224
    non-fortified, 105, 192, 223
    protein source, 181
    for tiredness on plan, 192, 223
Yogurt, 50, 128
    Greek, *211*
    hormone-free, 201
    sugar in, 110, 116, 172, 321
YouTube videos, 7, 223, 317

CONSCIOUS EATING
Cards

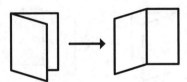

Cut Out & Carry in Your Wallet

• I MESSED UP •

☑ Consume 3 kale shakes the next day.

☑ Ensure your vegetable quantity is at least 7–10 cups each day.

☑ Keep up with your walking and/or exercise implemented for the next week.

☑ Take 12 Organic Cruciferous Superfood capsules for the next 3 days to support the liver.

☑ Take 9 Adrenal & Cortisol Relief capsules to add back in the natural B vitamins.

☑ Take 3 dropperfuls of liquid Trace Minerals for the next 3 days.

☑ Get additional sleep the next 2–3 days.

• CARBOHYDRATES •

☑ I am okay with NOT burning fat for 17–48+ hours.

☑ I am willing to gain 1–2 lbs from eating these foods.

☑ I realize my blood sugar will spike, then drop, and that I will start craving the wrong foods because of my actions.

☑ I am aware that the food I am about to eat will contribute to fat deposits around my liver.

☑ I understand that junk foods will cause vitamin and mineral deficiencies.

☑ I realize that I will gain fluid retention from my actions.

☑ I am aware that sugar feeds cancer and contributes to high cholesterol, diabetes and a loss of memory.

CONSCIOUS EATING
Cards

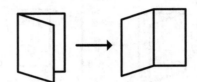

• HIDDEN CARBS •

- ☑ Sugar (brown sugar, maple syrup, molasses, honey, agave nectar, high-fructose corn syrup, brown-rice syrup, dextrose)

- ☑ Grains (breads, pasta, cereals, crackers, pancakes, waffles, yogurt—even unsweetened)

- ☑ Alcohol (wine, beer, hard liquor)

- ☑ Drinks (all juices, soda, Gatorade)

- ☑ Starches (potato, yam, sweet potato, french fries, white and brown rice, quinoa)

- ☑ Beans (they are mostly carbohydrates)

• ALCOHOL •

- ☑ I understand that all alcohol turns into sugar and causes fat to accumulate on my body and in my liver.

- ☑ I am okay with my liver being damaged and unable to burn fat for 17–72 hours.

- ☑ I realize alcohol is a chemical solvent that depletes vitamins from my body, kills liver cells and alters my brain chemistry.

- ☑ I know that alcohol eventually leads to ascites (fluid leaking from the liver into a sac around the abdomen).